Broken
Protocols

A Twenty-Five at the Lip
companion novella by

James Windale

ISBN-10: 1546670556
ISBN-13: 978-1546670551

For Kelsey…

THANKS TO THE FOLLOWING

Daryl Sugar
Kelsey Yahr
Courtney Garrity
Ryan Fraser
Michelle Disandro

i

The following story takes place
between Chapters 12 and 20
in James Windale's
Twenty-Five at the Lip

The year is 2007

SECTION I

Three jobs had come and gone since their seven AM start time. Their truck had started out with a respiratory difficulty out of St. Agnes of the Blessed Virgin which they took to The General. That was followed by the trip and fall over the steps out of a private residence that went to Union. Just as they were pulling back out onto the street dispatch hit them with a chest pain at a walk-in clinic. Calvin had given his standard "Walk-ins are for sprains and stitches, ERs are for chest pain and strokes," speech to the patient, but it had more than likely fallen on deaf ears.

They'd hoped to have enough time for lunch, but the coffee they'd picked up and done something for their hunger cravings. It was too early to eat anyway, and the only places open were fast food joints and hospital cafeterias. Jeremy had been making a point to bring his lunch with him, but that plan had failed through on the third or fourth day when he'd forgotten to pack one. Now he was back to waiting for Ming's Chinese to open up so he could get take out. Somewhere between *Stump the DJ* with Paul and Al on 94

1

HJY and a song by Alice in Chains playing, he'd dozed off. His head was leaning back against the headrest, dropping off to his left as it came to rest against the seatbelt swivel.

His left pants pocket buzzed, waking him up. He reached for the radio, Calvin still dozing in the passenger seat. It was a peculiar feeling, being awoken by something vibrating in his pocket. He looked around the cab of the ambulance, even watching the radio intently as if his superior concentration powers would cause it to make a similar noise. Then his left pocket buzzed again, and, he recognized the vibration of his cell phone. He flipped it open, a strange number beginning with a 774 area code stared back at him with a short message

Hey...

Jeremy didn't recognize the number, staring at it as his brain switched from sleep mode to full alertness.

HEY! the next text message insisted.

'Hey. Who is this?' he typed back.

Guess :)

He had no idea. Then in the pit of his stomach, something lurched, and he felt both hope and horror. He looked at Calvin again and saw that his partner was still fast asleep. Before he could reply with his guess, a photo came over the phone, taking up his entire screen. A picture of Carley sneering at him with her tongue lagging out of her mouth.

What's up butthead? she asked. At this moment he had the opportunity to ignore her and hope that she went away, but he also understood that Carley was not like her brother. If she wanted attention from someone, she was going to get it one way or the other. There was an opportunity here, but Jeremy didn't want to risk the still fragile friendship he'd been building with Calvin since their pow-wow in the Bohemian Bean after his near DUI arrest.

Jeremy had appreciated the attention from Carley at Dave and Buster's despite the fact that she had thoroughly trounced him in pool. She had been close to him then and when Calvin had disappeared to the bathroom she had become even more adventurous with flirting, to the point where she all but begged him to show her how to shoot pool on the table. When he did, she turned toward him, offering him the opportunity, but he passed it up out of fear. The little Grove Rat had been coming on to him the entire time and he'd blown it. He felt sick the entire way home, not sure if he should have gone for it. Waking up the next morning he'd felt better about it, despite the slight hangover he cured with a banana and Tylenol.

Now here she was again. At some point Carley must have either gone into his phone or Calvin's and found his number, saving it in hers.

He looked at the blinking cursor on his text screen and weighed the appropriate response. On the one hand, he could afford a little flirting, but the consequences might be dire.

'Not much. What's up with you?'

Nuthin'. I'm bored. Entertain me.

He cursed to himself. Calvin snorted awake, wiping the side of his mouth with the cuff of his jacket, and Jeremy's chest tightened. Calvin murmured something and opened the door of the ambulance, stepping out and walking across the parking lot to the Trucchi's. His heart was pounding he received another photo from Carley, a frowning face with sad looking gray eyes.

'Sorry. Can't. At work.' he replied. He watched as Calvin approached the counter at Trucchi's and placed a soda on the counter, fishing for his wallet.

K, well have a good day. Text me L8R, K?

What was she nuts? He could have let it go at that, seeming to forget all about it later on when he was supposed to, but instead, he chose to leave his finger on the trigger, just brushing it so that there would still be contact. 'K,' he replied.

He walked into his apartment, taking his boots off at the door and leaving them against the wall. Taking his shirt off he tossed it into the overflowing hamper in his already cramped bathroom. Turning the shower on and going into the kitchen to get a beer out of the fridge. Narragansett was his economic beer of choice and the sound of the crack as he popped the top was still heavenly at the end of his day. The sun was still out a little, setting in the Western sky over Segregansett and Ocean Grove.

HI! she texted again. *Miss me?*

He coughed and felt the burn of beer run up into his sinuses. He looked at his phone, the mental image of Calvin shaking his head in disgust Jeremy's desire to respond. Upending the can of beer he drank from it until it felt lighter, the shower in the bathroom starting to emanate steam out into the living room. Heck yes, he missed her. She had that tacky body spray the girl whose locker was nest to his in high school. Carley wore it too, and he never found it appealing until she wore it.

'Hey' was all he dared reply. Putting the phone down he stripped off the rest of his clothes and got into the shower, turning the water from hot to cold and trying to force Carley Peirce out of his mind. Stepping out of the shower, the ambient temperature of the room was warmer, and he felt better; a clearer mind and a clean sense of self. Starting to relax again he gulped another mouthful of beer and burped, feeling his body shake as he did so. With little food in his stomach, he was already getting light headed.

His phone chimed again, and he sighed, walking out into the kitchen again he picked it up.

What do you know about cable?

Basically nothing was what he knew about cable. He knew when he called the guys they came out and hooked it up. He also knew that his Xbox was running through it and that he was probably going to be spending the night playing Grand Theft Auto on it.

'Not much,' he admitted. 'Why?'

He finished his beer and tossed the unwashed empty into the cardboard box he kept his recycling in until he could carry it down to the trash. Carley fired back a reply immediately.

There's something wrong with mine. I'm getting the blue screen of death.

Jeremy knew that could be any number of things. She might have a loose wire or something like that.

Could you come over and look at it?

"Fuck…" he said out loud. Realizing he was still naked, but not because it was cold in the kitchen he hurried into the bathroom and pulled on his bathrobe, yanking the belt tightly across his middle. It did nothing to hide the fact that he was enticed by her request. There was that nagging idea though that this was all something he was imagining. He knew that Carley called on Calvin for lots of things that she couldn't do on her own and this may have just been a ruse to bring him on board with that. Hired help paid for with suggestions of attraction for him and family for Calvin.

Jeremy?

In a flash, he threw off his robe and crashed into his bedroom finding clean clothes to pull on. His sneakers untied he hurried out into the hallway letting his door slam shut behind him as he crashed down the steps.

Wrapping his hands on the steering wheel, he tried to convince himself that this was a bad idea. Carley was sure to mention this to Calvin, and then things would be weird between them again. Jeremy also figured that the awkward expression on his face was going to be a tell when she opened the door, and he feared that he might still be at half mast when she did. Visions of her recoiling at the sight of him made him nauseous. It wasn't until he reached her street and parked that he considered the idea that Calvin might show up at her house unexpectedly. Then how would he explain what he was doing there?

He swallowed hard as he raised his hand to knock, but the door was open before he could. Carley was standing there in a black and white baby doll shirt and tight jeans and no shoes. He felt dizzy looking at her.

"Hi," she said gleaming at him. She opened the door the rest of the way adding, "Come on in." She turned and walked into the apartment that he could remember from a few weeks previous. It was still messy, with vinyl records scattered around on the floor as if she'd spent the day just listening to music. Judging what he'd heard about Carley, this was not entirely out of the realm of possibility. The TV was still on and just as she had said there was a blue screen of death on it, signifying that there was no signal. He was both relieved and disappointed at the same time that this call to her house had been apparently legitimate.

"Are you hungry?" she asked from the kitchen. There was a smell coming from there that was rather appealing, and his stomach grumbled. He wanted to say no, but she opened the cabinet over the sink and retrieved a pair of plates from it. She had decided for him that he was going to eat.

"Sure," he gulped, turning his attention to the TV. He looked behind it and checked the wires, fussing with them and making sure that they were connected where they were supposed to be. All the connections were intact, and he even tried the input option to see if she just had it on the wrong setting. Everything seemed in order.

"I don't know what's wrong with your cable," he said sheepishly. "You paid the bill, right?" He heard the deafening sound of a large spoon dropping into the aluminum sink and Carley muttering something along the lines of

"Fuck a duck! That must be it. I feel awful for asking you to come over now," she said pushing off a stack of unopened mail on her table and placing the pair of plates down beside one another. They landed with a clutter thud, and she looked up at him again, grinning. "Beer?" Jeremy shrugged and then nodded and Carley went happily into the kitchen and opened the door to the fridge. She carried in a pair of Budweiser's and put them on the table. Sitting down in a chair she looked at Jeremy expectantly, the anxious young man not sure if he should or not. She nudged the chair with her foot, and he sat down in it, anxious about everything going on.

"Are you all right?" she asked.

"Yeah I'm fine," he said. "Just a little tired from work is all."

She stuck her fork into the bowl of casserole and started eating. Jeremy, not wanting to offend, did the same. In all actuality, he was so nervous that he couldn't taste anything.

As he left his heart was pounding, and his mind raced for what was appropriate at the door. He opened the door, and Carley looked up at him expectantly.

"Thanks for coming over. Sorry it was sort of a waste of time for you. I've got to be better about paying my bills," she said sheepishly.

"So I've noticed," Jeremy said grinning. She sneered at him and playfully jabbed at his shoulder, leaving her hand there on his jacket. Carley fingered the denim collar and looked up at him. He knew that he was turning red and she smiled at him.

"Thanks again," she said hugging him. She stood on her tiptoes, trying to get up as close to him as she could. He could smell her perfume, that sweet tacky aroma that had now been changed in his mind to mean Carley Peirce. Her skin against his cheek she could feel his heart pounding through his chest. Turning her head she kissed his cheek, hearing him exhale as if a relief value had let go. It was soft and wonderful, everything he'd imagine it might be.

Dropping back onto her feet she still had her hands on him. There was a look of joyful fear on his face, and Carley bit her lower lip, not sure if she had done something wrong.

"Thanks for dinner," he choked, smiling sheepishly as he walked away from her. The noise of his feet on the stairs was loud, and Carley stood in the doorway, leaning against the frame watching him walk away.

He slammed the door behind him, almost gasping for air, a full panic attack in progress. The day had been creepily surreal. Carley seemed to come on strong with so much of his being wanting to open up to her and let her in. Why though? She was not the sort of person that he was drawn toward. He was interested in women who were more academic that Carley put herself out to be. Carley was the kind of girl who had skated by in high school and most likely didn't have much, if anything, in the way of college credits? Did that even matter?

On the one hand it did because Carley was already barely able to pay her bills. If she had a job that paid more she would be able to support herself better, and that would make her more responsible and more reliable when it came to functioning as an adult. That was what his mother would have said though, and her programming in his mind had provided for that level of thinking when it came to choosing a suitable prospective mate. Tossing his keys on the table, he reasoned that he wasn't looking for a mate.

On the other hand there was no uncertainty about the fact that Jeremy found Carley incredibly attractive. She had a spirit about her that was both friendly and engaging. He wanted to be around her, despite nearly running away from her front door after she kissed him. There was no urge to wipe it away, and at the first stop sign he checked it in the rearview mirror to see if there was anything residual left on his face. He was disappointed to find nothing, only the memory that made his heart pound in his chest and the butterflies in his stomach. Now at home, he wished he'd stayed longer.

Then there as Calvin, Carley's brother. It was strange to think of him in such a way as it had always been the other way around. Carley was Calvin's sister, and according to BroCode worldwide you did not date your friend's sister. Acts on such levels were high crimes or misdemeanors at the very least. That way she felt though, leaning against him in the doorway, her arms around his shoulders stretching up to kiss him. She'd wanted more. There was no way she hadn't known that her cable was out, she had set him up. It had been a ploy all along to get him over to her house without Calvin around. He didn't know if he had survived or blown the biggest opportunity of his life.

Shutting his eyes, he tried to not think about her. Then, of course, everything came to mind. The way she walked and swayed her hips. It must have been deliberate. The low cut shirts, and the way she always managed to have her hand, arm, or something touching him. She had felt good, and he wished that he had reciprocated when she'd shown him that affection at the door. He tried to remember the smell of her perfume as he drifted off to sleep.

SECTION II

"Guess what floor Mickey lives on," Calvin said handing Jeremy the paperwork on the patient they were taking off the floor at Union Hospital. Hargraves 5 was the unit best known for bariatric care, or the patients who exceeded the distinction of morbid obesity. Most of them were there for various infections relating to their condition, as well as the typical ailments such as difficulty breathing, congestive heart failure, and other classifications that deemed them unable to thrive. Many of them had simply given up on reversing the inevitability of their health decline and ultimate mortality. Then there was Mickey Machado, famous on YouTube for uploading videos of himself dancing shirtless with his extraordinary amount of body fat hanging off of him. At his last weight he was reported to be closing in on nine hundred pounds. His rendition of Genie in a Bottle was said to be enough to make a weak stomach turn, but Mickey's smell was guaranteed to do that if his videos didn't. The smell is like a dank yeast. It lingers in the air or can play hide and seek with your senses as the odor escapes the folds under the skin. Once it hits your nose, you'll spend hours trying to get it out of there. It seems to bind to your nose hairs, clinging to you like a life raft until it eventually dissipates. The smell of death is sometimes preferable to the living funk of the over eight hundred pound crowd.

"First floor, with a wide wheelchair ramp and a crane to hoist him from our stretcher onto his bed or couch and then a full complement of nurses to settle him in?" Jeremy asked sarcastically.

"Close," Calvin said slapping the paperwork onto his aluminum clipboard. "Third floor, tenement walkup complete with narrow, winding staircase, rotten wood and as a bonus: German cockroaches."

"Well if we get stuck in there cockroaches are full of protein," Jeremy suggested.

"True. See you're thinking outside the box, that's good."

The nurse approached the edge of the desk, a pleading look on her face.

"For the love of Gawd, get that piece of shit off my floor," she said.

"That bad, huh?" Calvin asked. The nurse sighed and put her face on the desktop.

"It's not his size or even the smell," she explained. "He's an asshole."

"Really?" Calvin asked. "He seems so happy on YouTube."

"You'd be happy too if the state were paying you to be a half-ton load of shit," she countered. "He's on a weight management plan, but orders pizza to his room. There were two boxes stacked up on the radiator beside the bottles of Mountain Dew he's got lined up. We go in and explain to him, you know, in our best customer service way, that he's on a strict diet and can't eat that stuff, and he just goes off. 'Fuck you, stupid, ignorant bitch,' this and that," the nurse continued. "Finally the doctor told him he was being discharged. He doesn't want to comply, so he's being fired as a patient. Then it's a sob story about how he isn't being treated well. Spare me."

"Okay then," Calvin said turning to Jeremy. "Down the hall?"

"Just follow your nose, as the toucan says," the nurse replied. "He's got years of stink and funk under those folds; you can't miss him."

The paperwork tucked into Jeremy's back pocket they started the trek down the corridor. They wheeled the stretcher into the room, and the odor of Mickey Machado hit them immediately. He was laying in his bariatric bed, complete with air support mattress working harder than any other piece of machinery in the hospital to keep him elevated. Jeremy caught a whiff of Mickey, a mere thirty-three years old, with purple legs covered in scabs and dripping with pustules. He was busy working on a dinner tray, scraping the remnants of his cardiac diet into his mouth from his plate. This might have been a good start for him if there were not half a dozen bottles of Mountain Dew lining the windowsill.

"He shouldn't leave those out in direct sunlight," Calvin muttered. "He might get cancer from the BPAs from the plastic."

"I'm sure he would want to be as proactive about all that, if only he knew," Jeremy said.

Mickey returned the empty plate to the table and pushed the tray table aside. He wiped his face with his hands and then flicked at the crumbs littering his blankets.

"I'm going to need you to move me," Mickey said. "I can't walk."

"I see," Calvin said. "So you're not the guy who dances in all those videos on Youtube?"

Mickey's face shook, jiggling his jowls and unshaven face. Jeremy coughed, the smell finally getting to him as he stepped outside the room. The nurse at the station smirked at him.

At the end of the hall two more crews showed up. For his part, Calvin was relieved to see that Valerie wasn't one of them. They sauntered down the corridor, looking relieved that they weren't the ones who had to transport the infamous patient, only assist with the lifting on scene and at the destination. They were a pair of BLS crews, a pair of new faces to Calvin, and a couple of older ones as well.

"Short straw, huh Peirce?" one of them asked. He was a short and spiked hair gelled Basic EMT named Steve.

"You could say that," Calvin replied. Jeremy was busying himself over by the isolation cart, fitting himself for a surgical mask to cut the smell of Mickey.

"How is it working with this shit head?" another muttered under his breath. This one was called Anthony. He was short and muscular, the sort of EMT with a case of small hands wearing large gloves. Anthony seemed to swim in them, but he insisted that he needed larges.

"He's really great actually. You now how it is, Bobby Carreiro forgets he was a new medic once." He looked at them sternly, in only the way a Medic could remind an EMT of their humility. "You guys forget too?" They shook their heads or looked away. "Didn't think so." He turned back to Jeremy and reached out for the surgical mask on his face,

"Don't bother it won't do you any good. The smell cuts through everything. You just have to man up."

The six of them entered the room, and the smell hit them instantly. A few coughed, but Calvin could see Jeremy holding his composure, not wanting to let them see him flinch.

"Hey, aren't you the guy who dances on YouTube?" Anthony asked. Mickey shook his head. "Yeah, sure you are, I bet you can walk to the stretcher, right?"

Again Mickey denied who he was and the wide bariatric stretcher was brought up alongside his bed. The four who had arrived groaned with their eyes, rolling them while gathering the sheet from around the inflatable mattress. With three to a side, the three crews secured as much of the sheet beneath Mickey as they could, the nurse rushing in just as they were about to move him offering

"I'll get the feet!" In other words, 'I want to look helpful and be part of the team, but want to do as little work as humanly possible.' Sliding Mickey over the yellow stretcher groaned under his incredible weight. It creaked, and they watched in horror, half expecting the legs to collapse beneath it to the floor. The legs held, and Anthony, wanting to prove his strength began to pull it to the open doorway and into the hall. They paused at the twin elevators, pushing the button in the center of the wall, the light overhead dinging as the doors opened wide. They pushed the stretcher in, the elevator seeming to list as they rolled him to the opposite wall.

"We'll take the stairs," the other crews offered rather than travel down in a maxed out elevator. The door shutting before Jeremy and Calvin set the stage for instant claustrophobia.

They pushed the stretcher out of the elevator, Jeremy reenacting his own Israelite's experience under the pharaohs of Egypt building pyramids. Outside in the parking lot the three crews assembled and together lifted the stretcher with the wheels into the ambulance, sliding it in with a deafening thud. There was a mechanical winch inside the truck that would have made it easier to load heavy stretchers with patients of this size. However, the mechanical winch, like many important pieces of equipment, was perpetually non-functioning.

Jeremy found the truck to be particularly sluggish with the extra thousand pounds of weight. It wasn't just Mickey on the stretcher; it was the stretcher itself. The ambulance listed down the road, Jeremy riding the breaks down Robeson Street past the Tio

Joao's and distinctly heard Mickey ask if they could stop and get him a coffee.

The three crews struggled to find available parking on the street. Rather than pushing a one-ton stretcher up two blocks, Calvin flipped on the emergency lights and set the parking break in the middle of the road.

The back doors opened up, the three crews lining up on either side as they struggled to pull Mickey out safely. They hot-dropped the wheels, the maneuver adding more work and strain to them as the wheels and undercarriage landed against the pavement.

The stair chair the sat in the side cabinet of their truck was rickety and even a little rusted. The lack of care that it had been shown was a combination of management not wanting to spend the money to replace it as much as it was the crews disregarding their employers for absurd rules such as no hat policies and no pay raises. It was a vicious cycle and often the equipment suffered.

"The stair chair we've got was the same one used to cart FDR around in his first election," Calvin said euphemistically. Do any of you have a better one?"

"Who are you kidding?" Steve asked.

"We've got a people mover," Jeremy said.

A people mover was the polite term for what crews referred to as the *Shamoo Shimmey*. It was a large tarp with handles that crews would lift their patient on and carry them across distances, often used as a last resort to moving patients large enough to draw an orbit. It wasn't exactly designed to take people up flights of stairs, but it had been used to take them down from time to time. The others groaned in unison, some already stretching their backs.

"Anybody have any other ideas?" Calvin asked. When none of them spoke up he was climbing back into the truck and opening the squad bench and fishing out the bright orange tarp out and throwing it onto the sidewalk. The other EMTs looked down in disgust at what they were being forced to do.

"Look on the bright side," Calvin said. "The civil service test is coming up again next year."

Mickey was gracious enough to roll from the stretcher onto the tarp, though the stretcher had to be lowered enough to meet the level of the sidewalk from the street. Laying flat on his back, the crews gathered around him, three men to a side and with Calvin and Jeremy at the head they began their daunting task. They lifted him off the ground, the straps of the tarp stretching a creaking in their hands as it pulled tight under his immense weight. They heaved in unison, lifting him off the ground and putting him down on the steps as they hauled him.

"Ow!" Mickey screamed. "What the fuck are you doing? This hurts!"

"Sorry, sir," Jeremy said. "It's too bad you can't walk though. We have to do it this way." Calvin looked at his partner as if he were laughing through his eyes. He was working with four people who hated his guts, but he was keeping a sense of humor all the same. Jeremy was evolving.

The apartment house was three floors, but first they needed to negotiate the seven steps leading to the porch and the front door. On the porch was a doorway leading into the house, built as one might expect at the height of the Borden City industrial boom, the house was not appropriately sized for persons exceeding the weight and girth that nine hundred pounds demanded. They made the porch landing easily enough, though their arms strained under his weight. At one hundred and fifty pounds for each of them to lift, they were still dragging an adult person each up the stairs.

"Do you want to call fire?" Steve asked. Calvin sighed and stretched his back. He looked at Jeremy who shook his head.

"The problem we have isn't weight as much as it is logistics. We can call fire for the weight dispersal, but it doesn't solve the problem of bringing him up the stairs."

"What the fuck is he saying?" the Steve snapped back. Calvin leered at him.

"He's saying that you can call another three guys, but weight isn't the issue. Where the fuck are you going to put them? The staircase is three feet side. We can only do three at the top and three at the bottom at best."

"Fuck this!" the Steve snapped again. Mickey laid on the porch indignantly, a lump in the midst of his six handlers. Calvin pointed to one of the other four and waved him over.

"The three of us are getting the head and we are going to back him up the stairs. Watch the curve of the stairwell and be careful where you step, there's no telling how dangerous these stairs are.

You three are going to push from the bottom, one on each side of the leg, the third in the middle. You can draw straws for who gets the face full of FUPA…"

The stairs creaked as they began their ascent. Despite the cool air outside the stairwell was a sauna and sweat was pouring from them before they reached the first landing. The sound of the vinyl tarp, nearly stuck inside the narrow staircase with Mickey exploding around it, made a slow zipping sound as it made the difficult upward journey.

"OW!" Mickey screamed as they pulled him up onto the first landing. "I have a bad back you fucking idiots!"

Calvin resisted the urge to nudge the fatty corpuscle back down the stairs, mostly because of the EMTs still beneath Mickey, but also because there would be a lot of explaining to do about it. In hindsight though, his record was clean enough that he might have been able to pull it off and still get away with his job intact.

They took a breather on the first landing; Mickey wedged on the old, cracked linoleum floor. The six EMTs on the landing caught their breath and looked helplessly up to the next stairwell.

"Is your door unlocked?" Jeremy asked.

"Of course not! Gawd, you fucking people are stupid," Mickey blurted out. "My keys are in my belongings bag," Mickey answered. Anthony opened the bag, sifting through Mountain Dew bottles until he found a large keyring littered with obnoxious keychains and a single key. He handed it to Jeremy who went to the top of the stairs, finding a short landing with a slanted roof and a small door.

"This has to be a sick joke," Jeremy said as he opened the door, finding only a single mattress in the middle of the living room. The apartment smelled musty with moldy pizza boxes and Chinese containers stacked up in various places in the apartment. Jeremy suddenly felt better about the condition of his own apartment.

"How's it look?" Calvin asked as Jeremy came back down the steps.

"If you thought that last flight of stairs was fun…"

"Shit," another EMT muttered.

With a three-count, the six men began pulling and lifting the 900-pound wonder up the tiny stairwell. It was a symphony of grunts and groans, broken only by the sudden chirping of Jeremy's cell phone.

"Jesus, your phone has been blowing up lately," Calvin remarked as they reached the landing. "You been laying pipe or something?" They ignored Mickey's cries of pain and discomfort as they came up over the lip of the last staircase. His own discomfort was his own making, but Calvin kept that thought to himself as he entered the tiny, congested apartment.

Jeremy took the opportunity to look at his phone, the message he was expecting,

Hi! How's your day? from Carley.

Jeremy stuffed the phone back into his pocket, putting the ringer on vibrate. Almost immediately he felt another vibration and then another. He started turning red.

"You all right?" Calvin asked as he came back to drag Mickey into his apartment.

"Yeah, my back is just killing me," Jeremy replied.

He was inside his apartment no more than a moment when he heard a knock at his door. He opened it to find Carley standing there, leaning against the wall and looking at him sheepishly.

"Hey," she said. Jeremy sighed and opened the door. There was no avoiding her out there, and she simply walked into his apartment. He felt his chest tighten again, both wanting this to be a normal thing for her to do, and not wanting it at the same time.

"Hi," he said. Carley entered the apartment and shut the door behind her. She started taking off her jacket and Jeremy was dismayed to see that she was wearing a tight flannel shirt, the first three buttons undone, and hip hugger jeans.

"Gawd dammit," Jeremy muttered.

"What?" Carley asked smirking. Jeremy looked back at her, and she shrugged her shoulders, her chest bouncing in front of her. She giggled as he went to the refrigerator and got himself a beer.

"Nothing. This whole thing is just weird."

"That's what I wanted to talk about," Carley said. "I felt bad about the other night. I was just so glad that you came over. I felt like you didn't get it or something."

"I don't, just so we're clear," Jeremy said.

"What don't you get?"

Jeremy shrugged and remembering his manners handed her a beer of her own.

"What I'm supposed to do here. You're my partner's little sister. He and I are only now starting to be friends, and I'm going to betray him like this?"

"I'm more than Calvin's sister," Carley answered. Jeremy cringed at the name, and Carley took the beer from his hand and opened it for him, handing it back before opening her own. Jeremy looked at the open beer and the impression of her hand in the condensation around the bottle.

I can't help who I like, Jeremy," she said. "I liked you when you first came over with Calvin."

"Gawd, don't say his name," Jeremy pleaded.

"Why not? He's my brother," Carley said. "Is that it? You feel weird because he's my brother?"

"Sort of, I don't know."

"Well that's bullshit," she answered. "My brother doesn't say who I can date. I can do what I want and so can you. I've seen the way you look at me, and I know we want the same thing, so what's the big deal?"

Jeremy sighed, taking his beer with him over to the couch and sitting down. He put the beer on his coffee table and sat down, Carley hesitating before following him over. She sat down beside him, venturing to put her hand on his knee. "Too much?" she asked. Jeremy shook his head, rolling his shoulder over to relieve the sore muscles that Mickey had given him.

"What is it?" she asked.

"We brought a one-ton lard-ass up three flights of stairs today. My back is going to kill me tomorrow."

Carley shifted on the couch and faced him. She put her hand on his shoulder, seeing if she would let her. He didn't seem to mind and put his head back on the couch, trying to relax. There was a quiet moment between them, and Jeremy decided to let her hand linger on his shoulder. She inched closer to him, gently rubbing the back of his neck with her thumb while she squeezed his shoulder. He didn't flinch or twitch, just leaned against the back of the couch accepting her touch. She smiled as she started the hand movement again, rubbing Jeremy's shoulder and neck. In the quiet of the room she could almost feel the pounding of his heart through his chest, reverberating up to his shoulders. She tried not to breathe too loudly, worried that he might snap out of whatever trance he was in and stop her from touching him.

By the fifth single handed shoulder rub Carley managed to get her second hand onto his other shoulder. Jeremy simply allowed it to occur, facing away from her with his eyes closed and trying to not think about who was there. She crept in closer, her body nearly touching his. Putting one leg past him he seemed to glance at it a moment, but she put more pressure on his shoulders, and he sighed, putting his head back.

He could feel her breathing on his neck. Awash in her perfume, Jeremy relaxed into the comfort that was Car-, a truly shameful fantasy. Her breath was warm against his neck, and he could feel her thighs tightening around him from behind. Her hands were warm on his shoulders now, and he could feel her braving the approach oh her lips against his neck. She was close, but then she wasn't as if she was testing his reaction. Jeremy wanted it though because he believed that if he didn't know that it was Carley kissing him that he had deniability about the entire thing.

Then she did it. He felt her lips touch the crook of his neck, lingering there in a lustful truce between act and completion. He gasped and he felt her hands and body tense around him. Her lips relaxed with a succulent sound, hovering over his skin and causing the hair on his neck to stand on end.

She switched sides, one of her hands disappearing from his shoulder. He could hear her fingers working at the buttons on her shirt, the metal bracelets on her wrist clacking together. Suddenly the sensation stopped, and her hand was back on his side again, and she was kissing the other side of his neck. He let her do it freely this time, letting himself be drawn in by her siren touch. He felt her touch him, running a pair of casual fingers along the ridge of his EMS pants. Half of his mind was pleading with her to stop, the other side allowing his concerns to fall by the wayside. Meanwhile his body was responding the way it naturally should have. He put his head back, feeling the brush of her hair along his cheek, and the curve of her smile aghast his skin. Wholly hypnotized, she could feel her pulling him in, her fingers fighting against the barrier of his shirt.

He sat forward abruptly, suddenly feeling cold without the heat from her body against him. She had that look in her eye, a pleading look that paired with her unbuttoned shirt begged him to do it. She bit her lip and looked up at him, leaning back on the arm of the couch and brushing aside her shirt revealing the fullness of her chest which was held back only by a turquoise bra. She put her glasses on the coffee table and unfastened the top button on her jeans, the sound of the metallic zipper sliding down. Jeremy held his breath, seeing the yellow, laced panties peering out at him from the enclosure of her jeans. All he had to do was crawl into her arms and surrender. Her eyes pleaded with him.

He fell over the coffee table as he turned to rush into the bathroom. The beer bottles crashing on the floor Carley gasped, and Jeremy fell to the ground with a thud. The pictures on the wall rattled, and the old women downstairs had her fair share to say about it a moment later when her broom handle whacked at the ceiling beneath them.

"Jeremy!" Carley screeched jumping up from the couch. She ran to his side where he was holding his shin on the ground. Her boobs, restrained only by the bra that screamed for relief, hung from her open shirt. Her pants seemed to make no attempt to move, despite being undone. She liked her clothes a little tighter to show off her curves, but they were a pain in the ass to get off sometimes.

She'd really hoped that Jeremy was going to help her with that part.

"Are you okay?" she asked.

"Carley," Jeremy stammered. The moment was gone from his eyes, the trance she'd put him under was broken, but hopefully not his leg.

"Too strong?" she asked. Jeremy shrugged, and the ridge in his pants was subsiding rapidly.

"It isn't that, Carley," Jeremy said coming to his feet. His leg hurt, and he was already regretting the spilled beer on the table, but nothing more than the feeling that had been Carley's body against him. She'd been laying there with her shirt undone and her thighs, though still firmly in her jeans, pleading for him. Jeans were a thing easily remedied in situations like that. She was already buttoning her shirt again, a look of embarrassment on her face. She turned for the door, picking her glasses up from the floor. Her sneakers squeaked on the hardwood as she made her way back to the exit.

"Carley, wait…"

"I like you, okay?!" she turned around. She was beginning to cry, and Jeremy felt a worse pang of regret now than he had letting her off his couch without burying himself inside her. "I can't help that. You know the kind of guys I go out with, Jeremy? Assholes. I like assholes because they are cool and have nice cars and good drugs. But they treat me like shit, and for some reason I always go back to that kind of guy because somehow I think I can fix them."

She wiped her eyes, smearing the mascara. She sighed as it appeared on her hands. "I don't do this shit for everybody, you know," she said. "I hate wearing makeup. It makes me feel all girly." There was a pause as she tried to get the rest of it off her face and hands, finally deciding to wipe it on her pants. "I've had guys like you before, but I always cut them loose. You aren't like them though. I don't know; maybe it's because I know it'll piss off my brother, or maybe I like the idea of being with a guy who would treat me nice, you know?"

Jeremy nodded, not sure if he should speak.

"When I see you I get these stupid butterflies in my stomach, and you make me act wicked obnoxious. I get sappy thinking about you, and I've never been like that. I fuck around a lot, but you I actually want. I can't stop thinking about you, Jeremy. You don't know how many times I've wished I could hold you. I want you so bad I can taste it. What is it about me you don't like?"

"Nothing," Jeremy said flatly. "You're his sister, and that's the only thing that's stopping me from doing anything. There's a guy code that…"

"Oh, fuck your guy code, Jeremy!" Carley cracked back. "This is you and me, nobody else!" She snatched her keys off the table and went back to the door. "When you change your mind, you know where to find me," she said flatly before shutting the door behind her.

SECTION III

"Why are you so shitty today?" Calvin asked. Jeremy rolled his eyes and pushed the driver's seat back. He'd been quiet, the situation with who Carley was to him and what he wanted her to be had been wrestling around in his mind for days. She hadn't tried to contact him, which bothered him more. His phone had been strangely silent and devoid of her constant texting and calling. He suspected that somewhere there was a Verizon technician that had noticed the spike in activity to his phone, and then noted the sudden stop off. A microburst of female attention that had been Jeremy Young's moment in the sun. "Come on; out with it. It'll be like confessional; I'll even look away if you want."

"I'm Jewish, and you're not Catholic," Jeremy retorted.

"True, but you are what you eat, and Valerie was still technically Catholic," he said with just a touch of anguish. That one hurt, and Calvin knew he'd regret that later when he was recounting those events in his head. Still too soon.

Jeremy's phone vibrated again and he hoped that it was Carley. He wanted to recant his stupidity and take what she wanted to give.

He wanted to say he was sorry for making her feel the way she did when she left. Instead it was another woman from his past.

Big time paragod doesn't have time for his BLS friends anymore? Snuffy asked.

'You say 'friends' like there are more than one,' Jeremy replied.

Tsk, tsk, tsk, Snuffy said. *I'm the only one that matters. How is Little Hitler treating you?*

'Fine,' Jeremy said.

Hmm, something's wrong though, Snuffy said. *I can tell. Is it him?*

'No, not exactly,' Jeremy replied. 'Girl problems.'

Girl problems? What cunt do I need to cut for you, my love? I'm calling you right now!

'No!' Jeremy typed back quickly. 'It's a long story, but we can talk about it over beers tonight if you want. You up for that?'

Psh, I'm a good Taberport Irish girl, I am always up for beers.

'Okay cool,' he said relieved.

But you're buying and picking me up, Mr. Big Money Medic.

'No problem,' he typed before his radio opened up.

Attention Bristol County 458...

"458," Calvin answered picking up the mic.

458 I need you to take it downtown. 243 Williams Street. Possible stroke, on channel B-Bravo.

"Copy, Bravo," Calvin answered. "You know where you're going?" he asked Jeremy. "It's south of the highway down by Roosevelt Park."

"Yeah, I've got it," Jeremy answered.

"I'm going to let you run the show, all right with you?" Calvin asked remembering the deal he'd made with Jeremy. His partner nodded, and Calvin switched the radio over as Jeremy pulled into traffic. The lights on, Jeremy chirped the siren and putting his foot firmly on the accelerator the sound of the diesel engine whined up, pushing the truck forward.

"458 on Bravo," Calvin called into the radio.

458, 243 Williams Street. 73-year-old female with stroke-like symptoms.

"Copy," Calvin said again. At just past noon the sun was in the Western sky and brightly shining into Jeremy's window. Calvin sat back in the passenger's seat, adjusting the stethoscope around his neck. "So where do you want to take this lady?"

"Union is a stroke center, but Borden City General isn't. We should go to Union then."

"Good," Calvin said. "It's also closer."

They turned onto Williams Street and stopped in front of the house as a police cruiser turned the corner down at the bottom of the hill, speeding up to meet them at the house.

"What do you want?" Calvin asked.

"Monitor, oxygen, IV…" Jeremy began.

"Stair chair too," Calvin groaned seeing the steps leading up to the house. "We can't catch a break."

The truck in park they climbed out as the officer blocked the street with his cruiser, the blue lights flashing. Jeremy opened the back doors and Calvin climbed in the side door. He put the monitor on the stretcher and the oxygen and medical bags beside it. Jeremy pulled the stretcher out, the wheels and undercarriage cracking own as he released the trigger. Pulling the stretcher to the curb and setting the brake, Jeremy opened the side cabinet grabbing the stair chair while Calvin carried the monitor and the medical bag up the steps, leaving Jeremy the green oxygen bag beside his feet.

The officer was already inside, standing beside an old black woman. Her husband was sitting in the corner on the stool before a weathered upright piano. He looked worried, his shaking hands holding her medical insurance cards. The officer stood to the side as Calvin entered the room, immediately letting Jeremy upstage him with, "What do you want?"

"Hi there," Jeremy began. "I'm Jeremy and this is Calvin, what's wrong with you today?"

"She can't talk good," the husband answered. The woman's face looked frightened, the left half of her face tense while the right side was flaccid and loose. Her right eyebrow sagged along with the right corner of her mouth making her look as though she were a dual image of herself.

"She can't talk at all?" Jeremy asked.

"No, sir, she can't talk good is all," her husband replied.

"Do you have any pain?" Jeremy asked.

"N-no," the woman said. Drool was beginning to trickle out from the corner of her mouth, and Jeremy picked up both of her hands in his own.

"Can you squeeze my hands real tight?" Jeremy asked. As expected the woman's right hand was limp, unable to comply along with the left which was able to grip Jeremy's hand, squeezing it tightly. Her breathing cadence picked up, and she looked at her husband with a frightened glance.

"What do you want?" Calvin asked again.

"Vitals, oxygen, monitor…" Jeremy began hearing the oxygen bag at his side unzip, the officer beside him kneeling down and fishing around inside the bag.

"How much?" he asked. Calvin had already gone to work wrapping the monitor's blood pressure cuff around her arm, switching the machine on.

"Two liters on a nasal cannula," Jeremy said. The officer opened the clear packaging around the coiled nasal cannula and connected it to the oxygen tank inside the bag, the dial switched up to two. Jeremy felt a swat on his arm and Calvin looking up at him expectantly.

"IV?" Jeremy asked. Calvin nodded and directed Jeremy to the husband holding the cards in his hand. "What kind of a medical history does she have?"

"What do you mean?" the husband asked. Jeremy blinked and then repeated himself.

"Like, her medical history. Does she have any medical problems?"

"No, I don't think so," he said plainly.

Calvin interrupted, and Jeremy immediately felt his chest tighten. If there was something he didn't like it was the idea that Calvin had to cover for him. He immediately felt like after the call he would be reproached for screwing something up. This had not happened for weeks, but the feeling of failure still resided in Jeremy's mind.

"Are those her prescriptions?" Calvin asked. The question cut through Jeremy, and his ears and neck turned red. The husband stood up, nodded encouragingly and tried handing the list to Calvin who deferred to Jeremy. He looked at the list, seeing several prescription medications on the list.

"There's things on here for high blood pressure, high cholesterol, diabetes. She's on Digoxin too."

"Well she had those problems, but she takes medications for them," the husband explained. Calvin shrugged and went to work on the IV, while Jeremy connected her to the monitor.

"She's in an underlying A-fib," Jeremy said examining the strip that printed.

"We'd expect that though, right?" Calvin asked looking at Jeremy. "She's on Digoxin for that." The officer cracked open the stair chair and set it beside the couch while Calvin disconnected the leads from the monitor, setting the coiled chord in her lap and passing the IV bag of saline to the officer to hold. "Let's move her over. When was the last time you saw her normal?" Calvin asked the husband.

"About twenty minutes ago," he said as they slid her over onto the chair. Taking the head, Calvin wheeled her toward the door backward as Jeremy scrambled to pick up the remainder of their equipment. Awkwardly leaving the monitor and the medical bag at the top of the stairs when Calvin shot him an exasperated look, Jeremy grabbed the bottom handles of the stair chair and started backing down the steps off the porch and onto the sidewalk. There they transferred her over to the stretcher, the officer hanging the bag of saline on the stretcher's IV pole and jaunting back up the steps for the rest of their equipment while they loaded her into the truck.

"What do you want to do?" Calvin asked. Breathing heavily and beginning to sweat Jeremy ran a nervous hand through his hair. "Take a minute," Calvin said starting to write up the report on the run sheet, scribbling down the patient's name, date of birth, and address. "Go back. What have we done so far?"

"Oxygen, monitor, IV," Jeremy repeated. "Could do a twelve lead…"

"We could, but what do you think is more important?" Calvin asked. "We already know she's in A-fib."

"Shit!" Jeremy stammered. "We have to call report!"

Calvin nodded and then pointed his pen at Jeremy. "What do you think they're going to ask you when you call it in?"

"Time last seen normal, which was about twenty minutes ago," Jeremy answered.

"Anything else?" Calvin asked.

Jeremy's eyes darted around the patient compartment. He looked over the monitor and the vitals. The IV was in place, the twelve lead was going to be done on the way to the hospital. Calvin never grilled him on paperwork, and report writing was something he already excelled at. Jeremy looked up, panic in his eyes and his nose flaring. Calvin flipped open the medical bag, reached in and pulled out the glucometer, tossing it to his partner.

"Get a blood sugar," Calvin said. "It would be a shame if you activated the stroke team for a patient who was only hypoglycemic."

"Jesus," Jeremy muttered ashamed of himself. "Sorry."

"Don't be sorry," Calvin said. "Just get the job done." Jeremy wiped her finger with an alcohol pad and stuck her finger with the spring loaded lancet drawing a dab of blood out onto her skin. He laid the strip next to the dot and the strip drew it up, like a mosquito. The meter chirped and then a number came back; 103.

"103," Jeremy said.

"You want to call it a stroke alert?" Calvin asked.

"Yeah."

"Then make it *so*," Calvin said in his best Captain Picard. Jeremy smirked and switched on the airway seat radio, grabbing the mic off the wall.

"Bristol County 458 calling Union ER, priority one. Stroke Alert."

Union ER answering Bristol County, Code Stroke, came the reply back.

"73 -year-old female, left sided weakness with facial droop," Jeremy began, gasping for a breath. "Last seen normal about twenty-five minutes ago by her husband. Patient has difficulty speaking and flaccidity…"

Did you get a blood sugar, Bristol?

"Blood sugar is 103," Jeremy replied. "Vitals are 160/90, and rate is 130 in A-fib," he said looking at the monitor. Calvin smirked at him. Normally an interruption in his radio report would cause throw him off so wholly that he'd have to start over again. This time he didn't.

Okay, Bristol County, see you when you get here. Proceed to room two on your arrival. Union out.

"See? That wasn't so bad now was it?" Calvin asked.

Jeremy rolled up to Snuffy's apartment. She was already waiting outside, a white tank top under a black bomber jacket and loosely worn jeans and work boots. She flicked her cigarette out into the street and ran around to the passenger's side of his truck.

"Hey, handsome," she said jumping in and kissing his cheek. "Sorry, was I supposed to make someone jealous? I don't really have what you'd call 'girly clothes.'

"No, you're fine," Jeremy answered. One of the wonders about EMS is that it works wonders for breaking down social barriers, providing you're not a social misfit. Race, sex, and orientation only really factor in as much as you want them to. There had been a time when Snuffy would have been proud to be an out and loud anti-man dick hating bitch. Her time in EMS had taught her that none of those things mattered, and the most important person in your life might not only be the person you slept with but the straight guy you also called your partner. Snuffy had an even larger obstacle to negotiate regarding the closed EMS society, finding someone who was not only in the business but also a lesbian. There was the occasional curious girl who might like to test out the proverbial waters, but despite her best efforts, Snuffy could only make them stay so long.

"How was work?" she asked.

"Fine," Jeremy sighed. "I almost fucked up on a stroke call, but not really at the same time. I almost forget to get a blood sugar."

"Did he yell at you?" she asked accusingly.

"No," Jeremy said shaking his head. "He and I have a working arrangement; we're basically friends at this point. Well, not basically, we *are* friends. That's how I'm in this situation."

"Really?!" Snuffy said excitedly. "Are you joining the team?"

"What?" Jeremy stammered. "No. Gawd no, you know where that boy has been?" he asked. Snuffy guffawed, stamping her feet on the floor of the truck. Truth be told, she'd had more than one passing thought about Valerie LeClaire herself.

"So this stays between you and me," Jeremy said.

"Jesus, what is the big secret?"

"I'm serious, Snuffy. This is some deep, dark shit."

"*Arright arready!*" she said taking his hand and wrapping her pinky finger around his. "What's the big secret? Who are you fucking? Are you fucking someone?"

"It's his little sister."

"Whaaaaat?!" Snuffy exploded, starting to laugh. "Oh, that is fucking perfect! The guy is a total cunt to you for weeks, and now you're banging his baby sister! I love it!"

Jeremy sighed and wrapped his hands on the steering wheel. It was uncomfortable for him to discuss Carley with anyone as it was, never mind when the person was laughing at his situation as if he was in some sort of power position.

"What does she look like?" Snuffy asked. Jeremy sighed and passed her his cell phone. She flipped it open and went immediately to his pictures, where she found a gray-eyed girl with green hair staring back at her, smiling mischievously. "Aww, she's cute, Jeremy. I'm sorry I laughed."

"It's okay," he said. "I'm conflicted is all. Calvin and I are getting along really good, and next to you he's a really good partner."

"Next to me is good, as long as he isn't better than me," Snuffy said smirking.

"Tell me all about her," Snuffy said claiming her usual table at the Saint James Pub. Being the middle of the week there were fewer people, and the live band was substituted with satellite radio hits of the eighties and nineties.

"Calm yourself," Jeremy said. "What're you drinking?"

"What do you think?" she asked

"Narragansett," he said. She smirked and waved him in the direction of the bar.

Jeremy went to the bar and ordered a Narragansett for Snuffy, then seeing Magic Hat's #9 on tap he ordered one for himself, remembering that Carley had liked it at Dave and Buster's. It was headier than the Snuffy's Narragansett, but it held something deeper in meaning to him, and it made him feel better about the situation with Carley.

"So?" Snuffy said. "Is she any good in bed?"

"I don't know," Jeremy retorted putting her beer down in front of her. "We almost did the other day. I knew she wanted to, she was basically begging for it, and I almost went there…"

"Almost?" Snuffy asked with an air of disappointment.

"This is hard for me, Snuffy," Jeremy said. "It's been a long time since I've had sex with anybody and I feel like she has some kind of expectation. She's younger than me, but I know she's been around more than I have. I don't mean that she's a slut or she's easy…"

"But you think that she's been with guys who are better in bed than you, have ginormous cocks, and can fuck her retarded?" Snuffy asked. She clinked his glass with her own, following it up with, "Cheers, fuckface," and swallowed a mouthful of beer.

Jeremy blinked and picked up his beer, suddenly feeling extremely vulnerable and inadequate. He looked at the beer and felt sad, pushing his bottom lip out. Snuffy reached out and flicked his lip with her finger adding, "Put that shit away. You're not those kinds of guys, and that's why I love you. I guarantee that's why she likes you too."

"What makes you say that?" Jeremy asked.

"Because if she's been down that road before she might have had really good sex, but that was the end of it. Nothing went anywhere else and it left her feeling shitty. Trust me, I wasn't always King of the Bulldykes, you know. I dated a couple of guys when I was younger, I even slept with some in that awkward, 'Don't know if I'm gay,' phase. Most were dicks because they could be. I knew better though and I saw them for what they were."

"So what does that mean for me?"

"That means you have an opportunity to show her what a real man is like. She probably figured that you were a hopeless dork, yet another charming and endearing thing I love about you. You're also safe in her eyes. She knows that you're not going to fuck her over because you're Calvin's partner, even his friend. But mostly because you're shy and sensitive and eventually women want to fall back on a guy like that. Usually it takes them a long time to figure it out, I know my mom did. My guess is that Carley figured it out earlier than most women do."

Jeremy sighed. Sipping his beer and suddenly having a flash memory of Carley's cheap perfume in his nose again and the sensation of her lips against his neck. It made him think of his arms around her at the pool table when she played him for a fool so that he'd stand behind her and show her how to make a shot. It was most likely evident to her at that moment that he liked her, and not necessarily because of the pounding heart in his chest. Those eyes, those gorgeous gray eyes the size of dinner plates that pierced his soul straight through to his heart gave credit to her name, though he knew it wasn't pronounced that way.

"So what should I do?" he asked.

"What do you want to do?" Snuff asked. His reply was a shy smirk that quickly turned into a mischievous grin.

"Good boy," she said. "I think you should go for it."

SECTION IV

The sound of a banging at his door woke him from a sound sleep. Checking his bedside clock, he could see that it was after midnight, and he might have thought he'd dreamed the sound. There was a calm stillness in the air of his dark bedroom, but a growing anxiety began growing in his chest.

The sound of banging rattled through the wall again and he knew for sure that it was the real thing. He got up out of bed and went into the living room, switching on the light, almost immediately hearing, "Jeremy?!" followed by another round of nervous knocking. He went to the door and looked through the peephole, already knowing who it was going to be. Swatting the chain off the door and releasing the deadbolt he jerked the door open. Carley stood in the hall, leaning against the door frame again, but this time looking visibly distressed.

"I need help," she shuddered. Looking up at him, she looked pale and sweaty, her bottom lip quivering. He reached out for her, pulling her into his apartment, checking the hallway outside before he shut the door. It wasn't till the gust of wind blew past him from shutting the door that he realized he was wearing nothing but his Borden City Weaver's gym shorts.

"What's wrong?" he asked forgetting the deliberate distance he'd been putting between himself and his partner's little sister. "Are you okay?" he asked putting his arms around her. She hesitated before returning the embrace, finally reaching up behind him and holding onto his shoulders.

"I think I got drugged," she said. "I was out with these guys I know from Wintertide in Providence. I took a drink from them, and then I started feeling funny so I dropped it in the middle of the floor and ran out in the middle of the show..."

"Did they hurt you?" Jeremy asked. "Did they touch you?"

"I think they wanted to," she said beginning to cry. "Oh my fucking Gawd, Jeremy."

"What do you remember?" Jeremy asked.

"Basically everything," she said. "We were doing shots and then one of them handed me a beer. I had a couple of sips of it, but it tasted funny. Then this one guy, Chad, started feeling me up. I wasn't really into it, but then he got really aggressive. That's when I figured it out. At least I think I did. Do you think I over reacted?"

"Jesus, no," Jeremy gasped. He brought her over to the couch to sit down. Her cropped hair was a mess and her eyes were bloodshot, contrasting her fair skin. Putting his arms around her she leaned into him, holding on to him as if for dear life.

"I don't feel good, Jeremy," she said putting her head down on his lap. "Promise you won't tell my brother. He doesn't like Chad. He's obnoxious and flirty when he isn't plain handsey. Valerie slapped him one night when he touched her. I'm so sleepy. I couldn't make it all the way home. I fucked up my car I think too." she said quietly.

"I should take you to the hospital," he said.

"No! No hospital," she pleaded. "Just stay with me. Promise, okay?" She wrapped her arms around him and began to breathe as if she was falling into a deep sleep. Jeremy looked down at her, brushed her hair away from her face and then replied to himself.

"All right. But I'm going to sit here and watch you. If you get worse I'm taking you to Union."

She woke up with the feeling of sleep over her body. Her face was on a pillow with a familiar scent and she was confused as to where she was. The place was familiar and she knew she'd been in the room recently, but it wasn't until she sat up that she realized she was laying on Jeremy's couch. She was wrapped in a light blanket and still in her clothes from the night before. Her Doc Marten's were on the floor beside her.

She began trying to piece the night together, wondering how she had, at last, come into the home of her crush. Wanting to hear some music to drive out the thought of Jeremy from her mind she put on her best rocker chick garb and went out to Wintertide. Chad and his band friends were there and as typical she wasn't going to pay for any drinks, Chad telling the bartender that he was taking care of her that night. She had mixed feelings about him and knew that he wanted her, but there was that creepiness about him that put her off. Still, he'd never been so bold or pushy that she couldn't divert him. There was the beer he handed her when she was hot and sweaty. It looked fine and she hadn't thought anything of it when she sipped and it tasted flat... or was it skunked... she wasn't sure. The next thing she knew he was touching her, standing behind her and feeling the curves of her thighs over the front of her skirt. Then she dropped the bottle on the floor and started running, crashing through the crowd as her head spun. She rushed out of Providence as fast as she could, trying to get back to her own apartment before the drugs hit. As she came off the highway there was no avoiding the fact that the drugs were taking over her body and through flashes in her memory she could remember getting to Jeremy's house and then there was just blackness.

On the coffee table in front of her was a banana, four ibuprofen, and a bottle of Gatorade. A note was under the items and she picked it up, looking at the handwriting on it and the signature at the end.

Carley,

Don't freak out. You're safe. You showed up here in the middle of the night looking sick and scared. You said that someone tried to drug you, but that you got away before they could do anything. You were too far gone to drive home, which is good you didn't because your car is a little banged up already. You can look at it later, but for now eat this banana and drink the Gatorade. Both will help replenish your electrolytes, and the ibuprofen will help your headache which I'm sure is pretty bad. I'm at work till six tonight. Feel better...

- Jeremy

P.S. Please don't rob me...

She gushed; he was so sweet to take care of her when she was sick. Sitting up she could see that he was right about the headache, and she still felt dizzy. She wasn't sure about eating anything, but the Gatorade was the kind she usually drank when she was hung over and she opened it, taking a few gulps before tossing a pair of ibuprofen down her throat. Laying back down on the couch she felt her equilibrium return and she shut her eyes, snuggling up against the pillow that he'd given her from his own bed. It smelled like him and she wrapped her arm around it as if it were him after all.

The damage to her car was apparent. Her bumper was hanging off on the passenger side and the tire there must have picked up something sharp as it was flat and half torn off the rim. The headlight was busted, but there was no paint or blood scraped onto her hood, so she guessed that it was something concrete that she'd hit and not another car. She was irritated that she couldn't drive it with the flat, but it was an excuse to spend the day at Jeremy's.

Back up in the apartment she began fussing about, first by making coffee. Trying to sit at his table she found it sticky and loaded with opened mail, books, and half a dozen other things that surely had a proper place elsewhere. She assembled his mail, stacking it in a row and then placed it in the center of the table. All he seemed to have for cleaning products was Windex, but she made it work, taking the sticky film off his table and then finally sitting down to finish her coffee where she looked down at the floor, also grimy and dirty. Sighing, she smiled and knew exactly how she was going to spend her day. If he wasn't sold on her body, he was going to see what kind of woman she was playing Susie Homemaker.

After the Gatorade was gone she continued drinking water from the tap. The apartment coming into a semblance of order, the DVDs on his shelf put back together and the floors washed, she showered before doing his laundry for him down in the dark, creepy basement. Rushing back up the stairs she folded his laundry on his bed deciding to let him figure out where his clothes belonged. She thought it might have been too much to do his laundry for him, but it was the gesture that counted. He'd thought enough of her to make she sure was taken care of and safe so it was logical that she would return the favor. Even if that favor wasn't going to be returned in a way that was typical for her. Still, she took a few moments to lay on his newly made bed and wondered what it would be like if they were together. Just Carley and Jeremy. Jeremy and Carley. She grinned and looked up at the ceiling, daydreaming about him.

She showered and picked a shirt out of the pile of clean ones she'd washed for him. It was a Bristol County EMS shirt, blue with white lettering. She pulled it on along with a pair of surgical scrub pants he must have brought home from when he'd done his clinical time at Union. Calvin had a few pairs of them as well. She was finishing dinner when she heard the door open around 6:30 the night. He walked in, for a moment wondering if he was in the right apartment.

"Hi," she said suddenly terrified that he would be angry. Jeremy looked around finding his apartment cleaned and vacuumed, the clutter he'd begun to accept as home was now sorted and organized. The strange smell coming from the kitchen enticing, and Carley stood in the kitchen's entryway smirking.

"I was hoping to have it on the table when you walked in," Carley said sheepishly. Jeremy was about to put his bag on the dining table when he found a pair of plates, utensils, and a pair of glasses to go along with them. She opened the fridge and opened a beer for him. Not knowing what else to do he let her bring it to him.

"What are we having?" he asked, totally blown away by the fact that she was not only still in his home, but that she had cleaned his place and made him dinner as well.

"You didn't have much," she said. "But I defrosted the chicken you had and marinated it. I walked down to the corner to get come couscous and broccoli."

"You did all this?" he asked letting his bag fall onto the couch which had the throw pillows placed as if they had always been there. "You couldn't have locked up when you left."

"You're right, I didn't," she said. "You'll have to give me a key so I can lock up next time." She winked and pulled a chair out, presumably his and took the beer from his hand pouring it into the glass.

"Gram always hated when we drank out of the can," she said. "Force of habit I suppose." Carley walked back into the kitchen and continued stirring the couscous, shutting the flame down and waiting for the other shoe to drop.

"Thank you," he said. He started exploring his apparently new apartment. The bathroom smelled good and his bedroom was almost pristine. His bed hadn't been made in ages and the chair in the corner of the room now had folded clean clothes on it rather than a pile of slightly worn to dirty to filthy clothes on it.

"Do I have time to take a shower?" he asked.

"Yeah," she said cracking a beer of her own. He walked into the bathroom finding his hamper now empty. Dropping his uniform into the bin was somewhat satisfying and hearing it shut with a thump was unlike anything he'd heard in ages. His bathroom actually smelled good, like some sort of flowers, but he wasn't sure he owned any kind of fresheners. He looked under the sink and found a spray can of Febreeze as well as a Glade Plug-in.

His shower was clean as well, the Star Brite cleaner having scrubbed away the grime from the porcelain.

Stepping out of the shower he found his bathrobe had been washed and hung on the back of the bathroom door. It was soft, having been dried with a softener sheet. She looked out of the kitchen doorway as he exited and smiled at him before he went back into his bedroom. He found his clean clothes and was about to rifle through the stack of them before deciding that it might not be in good taste to disrupt the organization that she had brought to the place. It was a strange feeling having her in his place and doing things that a girlfriend or lover might do. He heaved a sigh, hoping that Calvin didn't have any knowledge of this.

When he was dressed he came back out into the living room, finding her placing chicken and couscous on his plate beside a pile of broccoli. She smiled at him, biting her bottom lip and handed him his plate.

"I hope you like it," she said.

"I'm sure I will," he said nervously. They sat down at the table to eat.

"So how was your day?" she asked. Jeremy coughed, reached for his beer and took a sip of it. "You don't like it?" she asked. Jeremy shook his head.

"No, it's great… Carley," he said forcing her name out of his mouth. She smiled when he did as if acknowledging everything that was going on. Carley wanted him to want her there and he was surprisingly calm about the affair despite their past interactions. The bundle of nerves he'd always been when she was around was starting to loosen up and for his part he was glad hat it seemed somewhat normal for her name to roll off his tongue.

"Listen, about the other day," she began.

"No," he said. "I'm sorry about all that."

"What do you mean, you're sorry?" she asked.

He took a breath and forced himself to look at her.

"It's been a while," he said. She smirked and poked at her couscous with her fork, working a crown of broccoli around on her plate.

"So it's not because you don't like me," she said. "Or because I'm my brother's sister?"

"You are your brother's sister, and yeah that's something I have to take into consideration. It's not necessarily a deal breaker though."

She bit her bottom lip again and picked up her beer. It was a nervous reaction, but she didn't care.

"I get that you're conflicted," she said. "I don't want you do be though. What happens between us is between us."

"Well like I said too, it's been a while for me, you know? You came on really strong and it was like every fiber of my being wanted you, but I didn't want to disappoint you somehow."

"Aww!" she cooed reaching for his hand. There had been touching between them before, but nothing like this. She put her hand over his and he laced his fingers in-between hers. There was a sudden spark of energy, as if they were meant to work that way. His belly did a somersault and his head spun a little. Her thumb stroked his and it felt natural and wonderful. "That's the sweetest thing, Jeremy."

"It is?"

"Well don't feel too inadequate. A little confidence goes a long way, you know?" she said winking. Calvin must have relayed the conversation they'd had at the coffee house to her and he wondered just how much he'd told her. He knew that she was good at digging for information, but how much she already knew about him from her brother was a mystery.

"I don't want you to feel pressured," she added. "Don't get me wrong, I want you so bad I can taste it. It killed me when you didn't react to me the way I wanted you to. Any other guy would have stayed when I threw myself at him. You didn't though, twice," she said. She looked at him and he seemed a little uncomfortable with her openness.

"No," he said shaking his head and turning red. "I've just never heard anyone talk that way about me before." Carley laughed, stood up and hugged him.

"Well you should have," she said. "Be honest, do you feel like you could have sex with me right now?"

Jeremy sighed. "Physically, yes. But I think I'd be terrible. Assuming I could actually make it to, you know... I would last about point two seconds. I doubt I'd make it that far though."

Carley pouted and then returned her hand to his.

"When was the last time?" she asked.

"Earlier last year. Well to be honest it was more like like two years ago."

"Two years?" Carley asked surprised. "I should just fuck you now on principle. How many people have you been with?"

Jeremy took a breath before answering, sensing that when she answered these questions for herself that scales would be notably different. "Just two. What about you?"

Carley puckered her mouth and breathed out her nose. "Promise not to judge me?" she asked. There was no way he could not judge her, but he liked her, so he hoped that the number wasn't astronomical.

"Yeah," he said.

"Three weeks ago, and I've been with twenty-three or twenty-four people," she answered.

"Twenty-three or twenty-four guys?" he asked swallowing hard. He nodded trying to process such a number for a girl two years younger than him. He'd undoubtedly led a sheltered life, but Carley seemed to have lived eons beyond his years.

"Well no, maybe it's closer to twenty-five or twenty-six counting girls too," she admitted. "Sometimes the line gets vague over what constitutes sex too; blowjobs, handies, being unconscious, multiples when you're the third wheel…"

"Jesus, Carley," he gasped.

"Hey you said you wouldn't judge," she pleaded. He shook his head.

"I'm not judging," he said. "I just don't see how I can compete with that. Those guys are probably ten times what I am. And I didn't realize you were bisexual."

"No, most of them are assholes," she said. "I'm not bisexual either, just frisky sometimes. Guys don't always know how to service a girl."

"That's what scares me. Not just you, but with any girl."

"You'd be fine, Jeremy," she assured him. "Fucking isn't what I want from you. I mean I do want you, like, I really want you. It's like you're all I think about and it crushed me when you shot me down twice. Nobody shoots me down. I've never really had to work for affection before."

Jeremy knew that was bullshit, at least in the sense of her family. Her father was most likely the cause for a lot of her behavior, but she seemed to claim her mother's family more so than her father's. Calvin was definitely an influence on her, and she might have sensed that his initial disapproval of Jeremy appealed to her father's influence, while his later approval of his partner tied in with the loyalty on her mother's side.

"You had sex with someone when you liked me though?" Jeremy asked. Carley shrugged and then nodded.

"It wasn't like that though. I didn't think anything was going to happen between you and me and a couple of days later I wanted you to come over to see what it felt like to have you around without Calvin. Total honesty," she said. "My cable's been out for two months. I owe them like three hundred bucks."

"Jesus, Carley," Jeremy sighed. He was stifling a nervous smile and wondering how this conversation was going. He worried that he might start to panic, or think poorly of this girl who'd captured his attention and his imagination, sending the whole thing into a death spiral. The fact that she was more experienced than he was really didn't seem like that big a deal. If he liked her, and he really thought he did, he would have to understand that she'd had a life previous to him being around.

"You know you bring up Jesus a lot for a jew," she said. He laughed, which made her happy.

"Okay, well, all that aside and in the past, I'm just not sure that I could make you happy. Like, sexually?"

"Give the circumstances, Jeremy, you haven't had sex in so long that I feel like I'm the one who has to make you happy," Carley countered. "The other night I was laying in bed thinking about all the bad stuff I want to do to you, touching myself and I'm sure the neighbors heard me moan 'fuck me geek boy!'"

Jeremy almost spat out the beer he was drinking. He was getting excited just thinking about it, and the anxiety in his chest was starting to change from fear to desire. She fixed her hair behind her ear and looked at him.

"That's really descriptive," he said.

"Well it's true," she said. "You made me masturbate, and no guy's ever really been able to do that. There's something about you that makes me want to be a better person. To be the kind of girl… the kind of woman my mom and gram wanted me to be. Honestly, Jeremy, those two girls you've been with; I'm jealous of them. They know you in a way that I want to know you."

"They weren't that impressed I seem to remember," he countered.

"Well I'm not them, am I?" she said bringing her beer to her lips. "And I promise you; they aren't me."

Jeremy blinked and stared into those gray eyes. For the first time, he saw beyond the alcohol, sex, and drug pixie quality that she put out. Inside there was a person who might be able to come down to Jeremy's level, or maybe it was the other way around?

"If sex is too much we don't have to," she said. "I don't want to screw something up between us. I know you work with my brother and that's a factor, but you and I are independent of that."

"I want that with you though," he said. Carley smiled and stored his hand.

"Well that makes me happy," she said. "We can wait if it makes you more comfortable though."

"Maybe a little bit," Jeremy said. "Let's go out on a few dates and see who we feel?"

"Like dinner and a movie kind of date?" she asked. "I've never really done that before."

"I thought you'd have been out on lots of dates," Jeremy said.

"Not exactly," she said. "Dates that guys usually take me out on are cheap and always end up, well, you know."

"Well I should take you out for real," he said. "Some place nice." He thought for a moment and then asked. "Do you have a nice dress?"

Carley's eyes popped open, and she began to revert to her pixie status. "You're going to make me wear a dress?" she asked. "Gram always tried to get me to do that. It's easier said than done."

"Try," Jeremy said. "You might find it worth the effort."

Carley rolled her eyes and stroked his hand again. "Fiiiiiiiiiine," she said. "I'll do it for you. But when we finally do have sex I'm calling the shots," she said winking.

When dinner was over, he helped her clean up, and they sat on the couch beside one another. He turned on the TV, and she put one hand on his knee and her head on his shoulder. "Is this okay?" she asked before getting comfortable. He nodded, and then she adjusted herself so that it was more comfortable for her. It felt good to sit with him now that everything was out in the open. This felt more natural than pining over him and having him reject her. All she had to do was be herself, and she'd won him over.

SECTION V

He met her at her place on the night of their first official date. Coming to the door with he could tell that she was watching through the blinds in the window, but she must have been nervous as he walked up the steps. He was wearing a blue buttoned shirt and tie with slacks, in his hand were a bouquet of flowers. Knocking on the door, he stepped back and tried his best to hide his smile as he heard a pair of rushing feet. Carley flung the door open and stood there looking at him with the famous Peirce grin.

"Hi," she said trying to look sheepish. He could tell she felt strange in the blue strapped dress that came down to her knees. She had ballet flats on her feet and was pulling at the dress around her back and her knees. She looked up at him saying,

"You look great, but I feel weird."

"You look beautiful," he said.

She grinned and looked at the ground muttering, "Shut up," before biting her lip and glancing back up at him to see if he was still looking at her. "And you got me flowers?" she asked stamping her foot. "Come in," she said offering her hand to him and pulling him inside.

There wasn't a suitable vase to put them in, but she did happen to have a new water pipe that she was able to fill with water and place the flowers in.

"So where are we going?" Carley asked putting the flowers into the water pipe. She couldn't recall the last time any guy had bought her flowers. There was the girl who had done it for her, Katie, but that poor lesbian had been hungering for her for some time before Carley had relented. She was cute in her own way, but Carley knew that she was only exploring her comfort zone and that Katie had most definitely wanted something more than just casual sex.

"There's a nice place called Deed's," he said. "It's really fancy."

"How fancy?" she asked. "Am I dressed right?"

He took the opportunity to look her over again. She was making his head dizzy just at the sight of her. He smiled and nodded. She looked amazing, a hundred miles away from the other encounters he'd had with her. He wouldn't have changed her if she wasn't, but he was glad to see that she'd made an effort.

"Fancy enough," he said. "It's the sort of place you wear a tie to."

"I see," she said approaching him. She ran her fingers around his tie and fussed with the pleat and the knot at his collar. "And you bring all your girlfriends to this place?"

Jeremy smirked, rolling his eyes. "No, not exactly."

"Well, then what makes me so special?" she asked.

"Because you're Carley," he said feeling his heart pound through his chest. She smiled, glad that she could make him melt that way.

"You look nervous," she said. Jeremy grinned again and coughed, his hands shaking. He nodded subtly and swallowed hard.

"I am," he said. "I've been like this all day."

She smirked and flicked his collar with her finger. "You have, huh?" she asked. "What are you nervous about?"

Jeremy shrugged and watched her seductive eyes tear his soul apart.

"I haven't been on a date in a while. I kind of feel like I went a little overboard," Jeremy said. "I know that's not really what you want to hear, but you asked."

"Not at all," she said. "Besides we've had dinner together twice already, and we almost had sex on your couch when I came over that night, remember?"

"That's not... that doesn't count... does it?" he asked.

"I don't see why not," she said. "But maybe this is our first official date-date," she said.

"I suppose it is," Jeremy conceded. "Sorry, I'm dying here. I'm not used to talking to girls. To women..."

"You're doing fine, Jeremy," she reassured him. She looked back at the water pipe and the flowers that he'd brought her.

"Thank you for the flowers. They're beautiful. I was saving this for later, but I might as well give it to you now," she said looking into her black pocketbook. Jeremy's interest peaked he watched as he fussed about inside the bag for a moment, only to suddenly switch gears, grab him by the shirt and pull him down to her level. She kissed him. At first, Jeremy was stiff as a board and taken completely off guard. Then he relaxed, putting his arms around her and pulling her close. He inhaled her as they embraced taking all of her in and wrapping his arms around the small of her back.

"There," she said as they broke away with a wet crack of moisture. "Feel better?"

"Much," he replied.

Deed's was in Providence, and that fact did not truly come into Jeremy's mind until they were passing over the bridge and they went beyond the exit for Calvin's house. She looked down the exit and then back at Jeremy.

"I think I'm getting that feeling you were talking about," she said. "It's a little weird to be here with you. I'm always going into Providence, but this time is different. I feel like I'm getting away with something somehow."

"Getting away with it would be nice," he said with a nervous laugh.

She reached for his hand a squeezed it. It sent a warm feeling through his body, and as she stroked his hand with her finger, he broke another smile. It was dark out, and that made things a bit easier. Deed's was in the same vicinity that Calvin lived in and Jeremy was starting to rethink his choice of venue.

"Don't worry about a thing," Carley said. "He's not out tonight."

"How do you know?" he asked.

"I texted him. Asked what he was doing. He said that he was tired and going to bed early. I told him he was lame," Carley said giggling.

"Why would you do that?" he asked.

"I wanted to make sure that he wasn't going to bump into us," she said. "The last thing I want is for him to find out about us."

"There's an us?" Jeremy asked.

"You better hope there is," Carley asked. "I got two offers today. I'm a hot commodity."

"Is that so? Two offers?" he asked.

"I told them I had a boyfriend," she said. "Hope you don't mind that."

Jeremy coughed, smiling as he glanced at her out of the corner of his eye. She was charming in a way that was equally infuriating. She made presumptions about them, but he was glad that she did. It was like she wasn't afraid to do something so dangerous as violating the sacred tenants of the Bro Code. Really though, it wasn't Carley that was breaking protocol in that way, it was him. He felt something stir inside him, like a change in his normal function that enticed him to come out of his shell. She reached over the middle of the bench and took his hand, squeezing it.

They pulled through the overhang of the parking garage at *Providence Place*, the Rhode Island statehouse only a hundred yards away. He was nervous again, and swallowing hard he reached for the parking ticket before snatching it out of the machine.

She hopped out of the truck, the concrete beneath her feet clacking as she came around to the tailgate. Her handbag was slung over her shoulder, and she was looking around herself, wondering how she looked.

"Do you mind?" he asked as he approached her. He dropped his keys into his jacket pocket as she looked at him curiously. He put his hand around the small of her back and pulled her to him, kissing her again, wanting to relive that moment in her living room before they left. She was bending to him returning the kiss in a way that made him not want it to end. Releasing her, she put her feet back on the ground, still looking up at him expectantly.

"You're teasing me," she said taking his hand.

"Maybe a little," he admitted.

The duo stepped out on the sidewalk, the city lights from refurbished gas lamps illuminating the new sidewalks as people came and went around them. She wrapped her arm around his elbow and leaned against his sleeve. This was a different feeling for both of them. For the first time, Carley was feeling important to someone she was interested in, and Jeremy had the same feeling. Pushing on the tall glass doors to a dark restaurant, Jeremy held the door for her as she slid inside, spinning around to grin at him as he came in. She hopped over to him, wrapping her arms around him and kissing his neck as the hostess looked at them awkwardly.

"Young, table for two," Jeremy said. The hostess smiled, took a pair of menus from the rack behind her and led them quietly into the dining area. It had a tall ceiling, with linen table cloths and napkins. Candles graced the center of every table and the people sitting at the tables were dressed finely, in suits and dresses, while a viola played hauntingly in the far corner. Jeremy pulled Carley's seat out, and she couldn't help but give the hostess an excited look as she sat down at the table.

"Jeremy," Carley whispered. "I don't think I'm white enough to eat in this place."

"Do you always say exactly what's on your mind?" Jeremy asked with a grin.

Carley shrugged, glancing at the basket of bread that was brought to the table. She picked on out and bit into it directly, the waiter withdrawing his hand from the table before he poured olive oil into the dipping dish. Carley looked at Jeremy candidly, stopped chewing, and placed the rest of her bread in front of her. The waiter continued about his business, setting their table up and reviewing the menu with them before leaving them to bring back a bottle of wine.

"Don't you?" she replied. The simple answer was that he didn't. He'd never been that way. He'd hated the idea of making other people uncomfortable and rather than allow himself to just act like an average young person. Instead, he'd forced himself to live like an awkward middle-aged man in the body of a twenty-four-year-old.

"If that's the case then we're both in trouble," he said. "But my family's been coming here for years. It was the kind of place that made me feel really stuffy as a kid, but now it's sort of appealing."

"I like that you brought me here," she said. "I've never been in a place this nice before. I used to think that church suppers were big affairs, and then Gram and Grampa would take us to these old people restaurants when we were kids. They were quiet like this, but they weren't as much fun. I think it's because when you're young like that, all you really want to do is go jump in the ball pit of a Chuck E. Cheese."

Jeremy picked up his glass of wine and Carley followed suit.

"To breaking protocols," he said clinking her glass. Carley snorted in laughter before drinking from her glass. It was an awful toast, but it was them, and she was glad he was playing ball now. He was finding it all right to laugh about an uncomfortable position, and she was melting for him.

"Church suppers sound interesting," Jeremy remarked.

"You didn't have those at the synagogue?" Carley asked. Jeremy shrugged.

"We identify as Jewish, but we only go to temple on the important holidays. It was more important when we were younger, and my grandfather came back from the war wanting us to really embrace it, I suppose. It got to be a lot for my brother, and he didn't really keep up with it as much as he should. I did a little for

Mom, but even my dad would get anxious about going to every service." Jeremy sipped his wine again and put his glass on the table. "You know what I mean?"

Carley nodded. She'd sat in the Old White Church during Sunday Services when she was a little girl and before the sermon would go down into the small classroom where she and her brother would have Sunday School. It was never really a huge hit with them, but almost anything would have been preferable when she was older. Calvin stopped going, but there was a sort of claim they both had to the church, and if Gram were feeling sad or lonely they would go with her. Days like Christmas or Easter were non-negotiable in their eyes, and then around their grandfather's birthday or the anniversary of his death. There were times when they wanted to feel connected to something larger than themselves, even if they didn't know exactly what they believed in terms of a supreme being.

"My grampa was in the war too," Carley said. "But he was in Burma."

"Yeah, Calvin mentioned that," Jeremy said. Carley blushed, bringing her glass of wine up to hide her face. It was a silly thing, but the idea that they were mentioning Calvin, he-who-must-not-know, was doing something to lessen the tension in their sordid affair.

"Were any of your family," she began to ask. He'd brought up the issue on his own, and it stood to reason that if his grandfather had been impacted by it that he must have. "Involved?"

He nodded. "I didn't know any of them, but my grandfather did when he was a little boy. By the time he went back they were already lost. We remember them in our own way, and to hear him talk about it can be upsetting. He wanted to make sure that none of us lost touch with who we are." He reached across the table and squeezed her hand. "So now I'm dating a Christian girl," he said laughing.

"Well like you, it's more of an affiliation thing," Carley smirked. "Do you think he'd object?"

"No," Jeremy said. "He's not that bad."

"I've heard stories about my dad's family," Carley replied. "My mémère and pépère would be very upset that I'm not dating a nice Catholic boy. Or a French Canadian at that. They're funny old people. He's gone now, but Mémère Robidoux didn't even speak English until she was eight. Her family were factory workers in Woonsocket in the mills. How my father met up with my mother, I'll never know, but I do know that I'm not the favorite granddaughter on that side of the family. There's probably a lot of reasons for that though, mostly because my dad's had a lot of problems and they think I do too."

"It's cool because I can see how you and Calvin are similar, but then there are definite differences. You have the same color eyes, but your features are different."

"Well I'm a girl," Carley said sticking out her tongue.

"No, I mean you can tell you're related, but you're different," he said.

Carley nodded, "We've been told that too. Gram always hated having to explain that he and I have different dads, and for a while, I was telling people that my dad was Calvin's because of the stuff I heard old people say about our mom at church. There was this one really old lady who was wicked mean, and said that what happened to our mom was God punishing her for being a loose woman," Carley said. She bit into her bread again and sucked down half of her glass of wine. That concept seemed to have some impact on Carley, and Jeremy wondered if there was some connection there, but didn't want to presume. He was with her and he was glad to be. She was special and being in that place with her was more than he could have hoped for.

"But fuck that bitch," Carley said as she brought her glass down to the table. It was empty, and Jeremy refilled it. Carley winked at him and the waiter approached top take their orders.

"Waterfire!" Carley cheered as they left the restaurant. "Oh my Gawd, come on!" She grabbed his hand and led him across the street, cars hit their brakes as they hurried across, disregarding the crosswalk that was several yards down.

The riverbanks were crowded with people, the metal baskets protruding from the dark water holding flaming baskets of wood fed by boats that polled themselves up and down the river. There was an eerie quiet about the place, a peacefulness in the smoke and music that serenaded them and Carley felt Jeremy's arms wrap around her shoulder as she leaned into him.

They walked up the bank, the old stone walkways winding around the river on either side. The city shut the streets down and walking access was the only available means of travel in that immediate area. Vendors were serving food, from Italian to Portuguese to Cantonese, all the flavors of Providence were at their disposal. She hadn't seen the bill, but she knew that it was high. They didn't have prices on the menu, but he'd assured her that he wanted her to order what she wanted. She'd played it safe though, ordering something that she knew she'd like, rather than being adventurous with something she might not. Carley wasn't taking any chances; there was nothing that was going to ruin this night for them.

They passed a living statue beside the Rhode Island School of Design. It was a gargoyle that stood as perfectly still as stone, then moved in great bounding steps before coming to a halt again like a massive stone bird, standing as still again as if it had been carved there. She pulled him over to the edge of the bank, against the iron handrail that ran beneath a bridge where a college student was strumming his acoustic guitar. She fussed with his tie before pulling him down, still standing on her toes to kiss him.

"Thank you for this," she said. Jeremy smiled at her, the sound of a log being dropped into the metal basket in the middle of the river catching their attention. Somewhere behind them, along the stone embankment, a girl was strumming *Take a Picture* on an acoustic guitar. Carley hadn't really thought much of Filter before, but now it sounded fantastic. A sight across the river caused

Carley's heart to stop momentarily, as her fingers grasped Jeremy's shirt sleeves. She looked back at him and gestured with her eyes to the opposite bank.

"Don't look now," she whispered. "But we aren't the only ones here tonight."

Jeremy looked up slowly, seeing a familiar form strolling along the opposite bank. Calvin was with a girl Jeremy recognized. Allison, or Alex maybe, from the Union ER lab. He was his normal aloof self, but she stopped suddenly, swung him around and kissed him. Calvin seemed to appreciate the gesture though and went with it. Carley snickered,

"That's so gross!" she squeaked. "Come on, let's get out of here before they see us."

It wasn't a planned thing, necessarily, but rather an unspoken understanding about where things were going. They pulled up in front of Jeremy's apartment and Carley was almost running up to the front door of his place, with Jeremy nervously following behind. She was clutching him as he slid the key into the lock, turning the knob and pushing the door open. Carley giggled in anticipation as they walked inside, shutting the door behind them.

"I have a small confession to make," she said. "I watched one of your movies the other day."

"What do you mean?" he asked. She winked at him, biting her lip as she unclasped her shoe.

"It was a dirty movie," she said. "I found it in back of your Xbox games. *The Seven-Ten Split...*"

"Oh shit," he muttered. He began to turn red and looked at the floor. Feeling the heat rise beneath his collar he felt embarrassed to hear this coming from her.

"Don't feel bad," she said. "It was good. Good in the way that porn in supposed to be good."

Jeremy looked at his homily couch and then back at Carley who was now standing before him with no shoes on her feet.

"Don't get me wrong, the plot was terrible and the acting was as bad as a North Korean propaganda film, but it got my rocks off."

Jeremy squirmed in place and Carley pulled the clip out of her hair. "Thanks for a great night," she said.

"You need to go home?" he asked thinking about where he'd placed his keys.

"Not until tomorrow," she said putting her arms around his waist. She kissed his neck and he began to tense up. Almost as quickly he began to relax, letting his head fall onto hers as he felt the warmth of her lips against his skin.

"Are you sure?" he asked. She nudged him back onto the couch and he dropped down. She reached for the wall switch and clicked the light off, the only glow coming from the light over the stove he'd turned on before he left. Carley hiked her dress up above her knees and climbed onto his lap. He was shaking again and she pushed herself against his body, kissing him how she'd wanted to all along. She wanted him to know that it was alright to do this and she put her all into it. She knew the kind of guy he was and she wanted all of him.

"Yeah, I'm sure, Jeremy," she said.

"I just haven't," he began. She cut him off mid-thought by kissing him again and then went to the opposite side of his neck so he could finish his thought. "Done this in a long time." He was nearly panting now and she could feel his heart pounding through his prim and proper shirt and tie.

"Just let me take care of you," she said.

SECTION VI

He woke in the morning with a strange sensation. There was a moment of panic, his heart clenching in his chest as the feeling that he was missing something important hit him. He bolted up in bed, looking at the alarm clock beside him reading 8 AM. Then he remembered that it was his day off, and he laid back on his pillow, breathing a sigh of relief.

She was gone. Jeremy realized that through the night she had been beside him and he could remember feeling her wrap her arm around him when she rolled over. It had been a strange thing for him. He wondered if it was some cosmic joke that was waiting for the other side of, but that never happened. She looked down at him, his heart pounding through his chest, and smiled. He worried she'd be upset about the trigger being pulled too quickly. Instead, she kissed him, reaching for his glasses as she rolled off of him and into the spot beside him. She put them on, looking at him seriously and said,

"Did you learn that last little trick from *The Seven-Ten Split?*"

"Oh my Gawd," Jeremy grinned.

"Hey, it's a decent movie," Carley said. "They found some creative uses for bowling pins."

Jeremy snorted a laugh. He'd thought about what he might do if he was in this situation, but none of that seemed to materialize. He thought he'd been frustrated, but it seemed like she was too. She called the shots, and when he woke up that morning he was sore, and even a little tired.

Carley stuck her head into the bedroom. She was wearing his shirt from the night before, with only a single button keeping it closed while she was wandering around the place.

"You hungry, Babe?" she asked. She already had a pet name for him, or maybe that was just a generalized term of endearment, but still, it felt good to hear. This wasn't so scary now. In fact, it seemed pretty natural. She put her knee up on the bed beside him and crawled across the comforter to him. Laying down beside him again she wrapped her arms around him.

"I could lay here all day," Carley said. "Mind if I do?"

"Nope," Jeremy replied.

"I was going to make you breakfast, but you seem to be out of breakfast stuff," she said. "Well, actually it more like the stuff you do have has this greenish-gray fuzz growing all over it."

"I forget to clean out my fridge sometimes," he replied.

"Sometimes?" she asked looking up at him. "Well, I'm starving. Let's take a shower and get breakfast. I'm buying."

He wasn't going to argue with that, and since he'd insisted on paying for dinner the night before, he wasn't about to tell her otherwise. She looked beautiful to him though, and as she rolled off the bed onto her feet he tossed off the comforter and followed her into the bathroom.

"So what are you going to tell my brother?" Carley asked. She tore into a piece of bacon, chewing it thoughtfully, trying to avoid the snake bite piercings on her lips. There had been a nearly chipped tooth when she'd first gotten them, and her grandmother, Ruby Peirce, had been present. She'd reminded her that such things were foolish to have in the first place and that she was ruining per perfectly beautiful features. Carley had been such a beautiful child, and if her mother knew what she'd done to herself, she'd be horrified. It was right around that point that Carley looked out the kitchen window and let Gram's words buzz around her, tuning them out and thinking about the Brown Bomber that she had in the cigar box under her bed.

"Tell him what?" Jeremy asked.

"About us, of course! After all, you've managed to seduce his baby sister; I'm sure he wants to know you've got good intentions for me," she said. Jeremy looked at her with a horrified expression, fearing that the girl he'd spent the night with had suddenly gone rogue, delving into his deepest fears about the consequences of violated sacred tenants of the Bro Code.

"Relax," she said. "I'm kidding."

They were in Bristol County EMS territory, but it was unlikely that anyone would put two and two together if they saw Jeremy with Carley. The downside was that if someone did see them and asked him about who he was with in front of Calvin, he'd have to come up with something on the spot. He wasn't accustomed to that sort of thing.

He sipped his coffee, shaking his head. Jeremy had broken a barrier even allowing himself to go to bed with Carley, never mind the idea of having to tell Calvin about him dating his sister. If there was something that he wasn't looking forward to doing it was that, and he hoped that Calvin would maybe figure the situation out on his own.

"Don't do that to me," he laughed.

"It's fine, Babe," she replied. "He's really not the one you have to worry about. It's Gram that's the real test."

The idea of meeting Carley's other family member hit him with a similar sense of peril, but she must have smelt the fear emanating off his skin.

"Don't worry about that," she said. "You're already the best guy I've ever attached myself to. She'll love you, I promise. She even liked Valerie, believe it or not."

"What was that like?" Jeremy asked.

"What was what like?" Carley replied. "Valerie?" Jeremy nodded, putting his chin on his hand as he wrapped his other index finger around the handle of his coffee cup. "She was awesome, honestly. I sort of hate the fact that I got so close to her now. I keep getting this instinct to call her or text her, like, every time something cool happens, or I see something I know she'd like. It sort of sucks now, you know? In a weird way, we were like best friends, except she was also fucking my brother. You'd think that would be weird, but it was sort of cool. I guess I thought that they'd stay together?"

Jeremy nodded.

"I actually knew her in high school," he explained. "We had biology together and she was always sort of a party girl. She was that girl who smoked weed in the bathroom and barely had anything in on time. I remember her trying to figure out how many days she could still miss before school let out in June."

"You might have just described me," Carley laughed. "I dunno, I'm mad that I lost my friend, but I'm also mad that she hurt my brother. I suppose I have kind of a fucked up sense of loyalty like that, but what you and I do doesn't hurt Calvin. It might make things a little weird for him, but he'll have to deal with it."

Jeremy shifted in his seat.

"Do you remember when you told me to ignore him because he's always moody when he meets people?" he asked.

"I think so, yeah," Carley said. "Sometimes things are a little foggy. I've smoked a lot of weed, ya know."

Jeremy rolled his eyes, smirking at her as she bit playfully into her strip of bacon.

"He was a real asshole when we first met," Jeremy said. "It was like he was out to get me or something. Everything I did was wrong, and even if I did something right, he found something about it that made all of that irrelevant."

"That's my brother," Carley said. "He's always been like that; periodically moody and quiet. He can be judgmental and mean sometimes too, and I sort of guess why. Our grandfather died and he had to take over a lot of responsibilities at a young age. I don't think he really had to in a lot of senses, but he chose to. Basically, he did it to himself."

"What I mean is," Jeremy began. He rolled his eyes, looking up at the ceiling and searched for the right words. It wasn't easy to explain to a, presumed, girlfriend that her brother was a special kind of jerk when he'd first met him. "He was really critical of me when we first started working together. It was almost like he was looking for things to gig me on deliberately. I figured out pretty quickly why when I learned that Valerie had switched shifts. I guess they thought nobody knew about them, but even I know that there are no real secrets in EMS. Everybody knows everything, and those two were as subtle as a hand grenade."

"Yeah, they were lousy with chemistry," Carley said. "It was weird because, knowing my brother, I knew that he was investing more in her than she was in him. Valerie was easy to get along with, and I figured that maybe if I was friends with her that she'd feel better about committing to him somehow? It might sound stupid, but there were times I know he felt like a third wheel."

"It was Valerie that got him talking to me, in a sense. He ran out of Saint James Pub one night in March, and I bumped into him in the parking lot. I convinced him to let me bring him to get coffee because he shouldn't have been driving, and that was when we actually started getting to know each other."

"That must have been the night," Carley started. She looked down at her placemat and the plate of food in front of her. "He'd called me asking what I was doing. I hated myself for it after because I heard what happened."

"What do you mean?" Jeremy asked.

"He saw Valerie go off with that guy. He didn't even want to go to that stupid party at Saint James. He called and asked me what I was doing and I told him I was going to some concert, but really he was just bringing me down so much I couldn't bear to be around him anymore. I hated myself after that because I didn't know how badly she'd hurt him there. He's an ass, but he's my brother too."

She moved her eggs around on her plate with a fork, her rye toast dryer than she liked, and there wasn't enough butter saturated into it, the way her grandfather had made it for her when she was little.

"I'm glad that you two are friends now, though," she said. "It's selfish, but I think he needs more friends. Calvin craves that sort of thing, but he doesn't say anything about it. He just keeps his mouth shut and goes out of his way for other people all the time. He's a doormat, and sometimes he does things outside of his own interest thinking he's making people happy and doing something good."

"And now he's a new sort of doormat?" Jeremy asked.

"Because of us?" Carley asked.

"Well I did have to be friends to be dating his sister after all," Jeremy replied. Carley grinned and leaned across the table, upsetting the knife and fork near his plate and planting a solid kiss on his face.

"So we are official then?" Carley asked. Jeremy nodded.

"Yeah, I guess we are."

SECTION VII

"What are you thinking?" Calvin asked. Jeremy looked at the 12-lead the monitor had printed. There was elevation in the anterior leads, but it was only in the AVF lead. Without an additional lead in elevation he couldn't call an STEMI alert, or ST Elevation Myocardial Infarction. However, lead V4 was also elevated, and he squinted looking at V3, which seemed to ride the line from one cycle to the next.

"I'll call it," Jeremy said. Calvin sniffed, looking at the IV bag hanging from the ceiling. He grinned, watching the drip set drop the saline into the chamber and down the line.

"Good call," Calvin said. "So what next?"

"We've already given one nitro, and he's due for another," Jeremy said.

"Cool. Ask him," Calvin coaxed.

"How's your chest pain now?" Jeremy asked. "From zero to ten."

The man thought a moment, touching his chest between the leads attached to it and sending the signals back to the monitor. He'd been clammy, with cold skin and an elevated blood pressure when they'd gotten to him. The garage he'd been renting was cramped and the recliner he'd been sitting in was in between a daybed and a work bench. The television had been on; The Price is Right playing in the background. He'd been sipping on a can of Natural Ice at 11 AM and smelled as though he hadn't bathed in a day or more.

"It's, like, a four now," he said. "Originally it had started at a seven, but with one nitro on board already they'd managed to knock it down. Jeremy uncapped the spray bottle and gestured to the man to lift his tongue to the roof of his mouth. He squirted the mist under his tongue and the man closed his mouth.

"The stuff tastes funny," he said.

"It might give you a little headache," Jeremy reminded him.

"So you good?" Calvin asked. "We should get going if you're going to call this a STEMI alert."

"Yeah, we can go. If he's at max dilation I'll switch to morphine," Jeremy said. "Union is where we're going."

"No!" the man said turning around. "No morphine! I'm in recovery."

"Recovery?" Calvin asked. "For what?"

"Heroin," the man said. "I'm also HIV positive."

Calvin looked at Jeremy and blinked, sending an unspoken message of mild frustration that he'd left that part out of his medical history.

"He's on Atripla," Jeremy said posting to the medication list. "I knew."

"Really?" Calvin said. "Nicely done. Okay, let's go," he said shutting the side door.

Jeremy slid back over to the airway seat and unclipped the radio from its holster and switched the channel to Union's frequency.

"Bristol County 442 calling Union ER," he said. There was a moment of delay before a woman's voice answered. It had a sweet tone to it and could have only been Ashley, one of the RNs in the department, on the other end.

"442 in route with a STEMI alert. Pain began thirty minutes ago. 324 milligrams of aspirin on board and two nitros with IV access. We are forgoing morphine administration due to patient refusal of narcotic administration. Vitals are 180/70, is 90, respirations are 18 with oxygen via nasal cannula and saturation is at 98 percent. We are four minutes out. How do you copy?"

Ashley was back immediately, repeating his transmission before finishing with, *"We'll see you in four."*

Calvin had the siren on, running hot across the city with a STEMI alert that didn't have any morphine on board. It was a deviation of protocol, but Dr. Sucre would understand, not to mention it was already on the recorded radio line. He glanced into the back to see how Jeremy was getting along. He had slid over to the bench and was looking at the cardiac monitor on the back of the stretcher, angled so that he could see it.

"You knew I had HIV before I told you?" the man asked. Jeremy nodded.

"I recognized the drug you were on," he said. "It's pretty new. Not sure what made me think of it, but it stood out. I also found your veins difficult to get an IV into, so that also tipped me off."

"I've been clean for a year, and going to meetings. I have Hep C too," he explained. "Sometimes you don't know how someone is going to react. Back in the day, it was the fags who got the AIDS, but now it's a lot of drug addicts. Anyway, that's how I got it, from sharing needles."

Jeremy pulled his booted foot over his right knee and leaned back against the wall of the ambulance. The man looked like a drug addict and must have felt that drinking a beer wasn't as bad as heroin, and he was probably correct in that. But alcohol could interfere with the way his medications worked, and judging by the stack of meds on the shelf of his little garage home, he guessed that he didn't have much going on in the way of happiness to begin with.

"The thing is," Jeremy explained. "We need to know what sort of medical history you have. It's not because we're nosey, or that we're judging you. It's because we have medications that can interfere with what you're already on and that can be really bad when you get to the hospital because they have even more advanced stuff that can end up hurting you it reacts with your medications."

"I just don't want to be judged by man," he said. "Only God can judge me."

Jeremy nodded.

"I wouldn't worry too much about God's judgment," he said. "You're doing the right thing by staying clean. You go to your meetings and you got help when you needed it. Just keep it up and your life will only get better."

"Amen, brother," he said. "Do you know The Lord?"

"Yeah," Jeremy said.

"I mean, have you been Washed in the Blood of Christ?" he asked. "Do you follow Jesus Christ?"

Jeremy smiled back awkwardly at his patient. There was nothing quite so sanctified as a recovering addict who was working the program. Being from a Jewish family, Jeremy naturally hadn't been brought up worshiping Jesus Christ. Then again, his family was about as Jewish as your averaging non-practicing Catholic.

"Sure do," Jeremy said.

Calvin's phone buzzed. He looked at it and then rolled his eyes.

"What does she want now?" he groaned. Jeremy was pulling his backpack off the truck, slinging it over his shoulder. He adjusted his glasses nervously as he glanced at the screen of Calvin's phone, the name *Carley* on the screen.

Sitting at St. James by myself, she wrote. *You boys should come hang out with me.*

It had been a long day, but there were a few things worse than getting a beer at a favorite local watering hole. Jeremy checked the screen of his phone quickly, seeing a text from Carley as well.

;) was all she'd written.

"You want to go get a beer?" Calvin asked. "Carley is at St. James."

"Sure," Jeremy answered wondering if it came off as too eager. Calvin hadn't seemed to notice, but if there was something he didn't to want to do, it was hang around the base after his shift was over. "I'll meet you over there."

Jeremy was glad for the opportunity to prepare himself for seeing Carley with Calvin along for the ride. He did wish that she'd told him ahead of time, but it had been two days since he'd seen her and he was missing her already. In the weeks that they had been running around together they had been careful, but Jeremy was feeling like he was living in two worlds that could never collide. Pulling out of the lot he wrung his hands around the steering wheel, hoping that this wasn't the start of a major disaster.

It was a little strange to see Calvin get out of his car at St. James again. He seemed to pause, waiting at the door for Jeremy as if he didn't want to go in. His hands were in his pockets and the sun was going down in the west over his home town. He looked at it as if pondering something greater. That seemed to be his natural state of being.

"You all right?" Jeremy asked as he came up.

"Just thinking about the last time I was here," Calvin admitted. "That was a rough night."

"Yeah," Jeremy agreed. "A little. This is a different day though. That day is gone and it won't be back."

Calvin nodded. He had to agree with that sentiment, though he wondered what it would be like to see that spot Valerie had been sitting in when she pushed her 'new friend' into fifth gear. If he went in now, it would be a fresh experience, which hopefully would not be encumbered by her memory. It was funny how so many places could be haunted by memories.

"Come on," Jeremy said opening the door. "You can buy me a beer."

"And probably Carley too," Calvin said. "She never has any fucking money." Jeremy snorted; it was true.

They went into the basement, following the carpeted stairs flanked by brick walls. There was no band this evening, only the satellite radio playing 90s hits, which settled Calvin's mind better.

Carley was alone at a bar table, sitting high up with a half glass of beer in front of her. She smiled at Calvin and Jeremy as they walked in, their white uniform shirts off, and only the navy blue tee shirt they wore beneath left. It was their place in many ways though, and Bristol County EMS was known to use it as a hangout, not to mention the Borden City police and fire departments.

"Hey," she said to Calvin as he came up. Jeremy pulled a stool out across from her as Calvin picked one beside his sister. Her clothing choices were a far cry from the night at Dave and Buster's. A flannel patterned short-sleeved shirt, with a black tee beneath. Her jeans were modest, and if she'd wanted to play things cool, she was certainly pulling it off.

"'Sup?" Calvin replied. "What'd you get?"

"Number 9," Carley answered. "You have to order from the bar though, the wait staff isn't here in the afternoon. I sat here for, like, ten minutes before the told me."

"Unbelievable. This place has really gone downhill,"Calvin said smirking. It might have been a strange occurrence for his sister to actually have to go to the bar and order a beer, but most guys had to do that on the regular. "What are you drinking?" He asked Jeremy.

"Number 9," Jeremy said.

"Poser," he said.

"You're buying," Jeremy reminded him.

"I know, I know," Calvin said as he went to the bar. Carley watched him as he walked off, leaning on the counter looking at the chalkboard prices behind the bar before she leaned over quickly, grabbing Jeremy across the table by his shirt and pulling him toward her. She kissed him quickly, releasing him back to his seat.

"Hi, handsome," she whispered smirking.

"Hi," he said feeling the heat beneath his collar come to a flash point. He was on the verge of a panic, but Calvin hadn't seen a thing, only leaned against the bar, waiting for the bartender to come from the back room again. "Beautiful," he finished.

"You're sweet," she said.

"What are we doing?" he asked. It seemed like a crazy idea to have them together in front of Calvin, who wasn't supposed to know anything about them.

"We're keeping up appearances," she said. "Besides, this might be good in a way. If he gets used to the idea of seeing us together it might not be a big deal in the end."

"Its a good idea," Jeremy conceded. "But I hate not being able to be normal with you. It's like I've crossed some kind of point of no return and I don't want to just be your friend. I want more. I want all of you."

Her eyes widened and she bit her lip. Checking behind her she could still see her brother waiting for the bartender to come out from the back. The man showed, and Calvin got his attention. Carley reached across the table and squeezed Jeremy's hand.

"Come over later," she said. "Drive around the block until you lose him and then come straight to my place."

Jeremy grinned. It was a good plan, and it made sense. There was something about sneaking around that appealed to him. Though they were breaking fundamental rules, they weren't doing anything especially wrong in the grand scheme of things. Besides, Calvin had broken a similar rule with Valerie, though his outcome had been dramatically different than theirs.

He came back around with their beers, sliding Jeremy's over to him as Carley did her best to avoid the obvious chemistry that she'd been having with her brother's friend.

"Did Gram call you?" Carley asked. "She wanted to know if you were coming over on Saturday for supper."

"What is she making?" Calvin asked. It didn't matter what she was making, Calvin would be there regardless. He always went early too, because Ruby Peirce always had a to-do list for her grandson.

"Seafood casserole," she said. "The one with the Ritz Crackers and the spicy chili powder." Then as if it came out of nowhere, Carley had a brilliant idea. "Ohmigosh, Jeremy, you should totally come over our Gram's for dinner."

He was halfway through a sip of his beer and nearly expelled it from his mouth. He swallowed hard, looking at her and her dual snakebite lip piercings.

"You know how Gram gets," Calvin said. "If she hasn't planned on other people she's going to lose her mind."

Jeremy interjected, looking to put the issue to bed.

"My aunt Muriel is coming for dinner at my parent's," he said. "Shabbos."

"See? He can't go anyway," Calvin said. "Not that you're not welcome," he clarified. "Ruby tends to get excited if there are unplanned guests or whatever."

Carley shrugged.

"She's always been like that," Calvin continued. "We never had friends over growing up."

"You had Valerie over all the time," Carley interjected. Jeremy picked up his glass, bringing it to his mouth as he began to swallow his beer in large gulps. Calvin looked at his sister crookedly before she continued her . "…and Jane."

"That was different," Calvin said. "I was dating them. I ain't fucking Jeremy."

"You wish," Carley said. Jeremy put his glass down again, a full two dollars and fifty cents of it consumed as the foam ran down the edges of the glass. Carley was leaning on the table, her elbow and hand propping her face up as she poked her tongue against the wall of her cheek, looking at Jeremy provokingly. She winked at him, Calvin unaware of her gestures toward his friend.

As if knowing she was being spoken about, Calvin's phone began to ring.

"Speak of the devil," he said picking it up. "Hey, Gram," he said.

'Hey yourself,' she said smartly reminding him of proper English. Calvin rolled his eyes, picking up his beer again for another sip. *'Where are you?'* She must have heard the background music.

"I'm out with Jeremy," he said. "We're getting a beer with Carley."

'Really,' she said. *'Well don't drink too much.'*

"We won't," he assured her, taking a sip hearty enough to polish off his beer.

'Now, Calvin,' she said. *'Are you coming over for supper on Saturday?'* Of course he was coming over, he wasn't about to pass up a free meal.

"Yeah," he said. There was a moment of pause on the other end of the line. "Yes," he clarified.

'All right, I just wanted to know. Also,' she said. *'I need the old refrigerator taken out of the basement and put by the street. The town is coming to pick it up Monday morning.'*

"I don't think I can lug a refrigerator up out of the basement on my own," Calvin said. "Did they say they'd take it out if you wanted?"

'No, that's why I'm asking you,' she replied dryly.

"Hold on," Calvin said. He looked at Jeremy, holding his hand over the phone. "You want to make some money?"

"Hmm?" Jeremy asked.

"My grandmother has a refrigerator in the basement that needs to go out to the curb before Monday. Do you think you could come out to Ocean Grove on Sunday and help me pull it out of the basement?" he asked. As if to sweeten the deal he added, "I'll pay you."

"Yeah, all right," Jeremy said. "You don't have to pay me though."

"You're not doing this for nothing," Calvin replied.

"Will work for beer," Jeremy said. He glanced at Carley who was looking at him lovingly. She was smitten at that moment, and suddenly what Carley had done seemed to make a whole lot of sense. "In fact, I can do it on Saturday if you want."

"But your Aunt Muriel," Calvin said. "Shabbos?" Jeremy shook his head.

"Eh, we're not that Jewish," Jeremy replied in his best Woody Allen.

Carley's broken-looking car was parked out in front of her grandmother's house when Jeremy came around the corner. He hadn't been here before, but it looked just as Carley had described it. He put his truck into park, looking around for Calvin's car, but it looked as though he was early.

Carley was walking around from the back step as he got out, hurrying up to him before Calvin made an appearance.

"He's at the packey," Carley said. "We've got a minute before he gets here." She jumped onto him, wrapping her arms and legs around his torso, kissing him.

"What's a packey?" Jeremy asked.

Carley looked at him funny. "You mean you grew up in Borden City and don't know what a package store is?" Jeremy shook his head.

"Kiss me again and I'll tell you," she sighed, holding onto him. He did as he was instructed, and she seemed to inhale him. "Back in the day, when alcohol was illegal, people used to call them packages. Gram's father used to say, 'Oh I got a package down in Bunktown.' That's where they used to run booze into Ocean Grove. It's kind of a stupid expression, and even a little white trashy, but I like it."

"It's not trashy," Jeremy said. "Especially not if you like it."

"Come on, come meet Gram," Carley said climbing down. She led him to the house, the shale rock way leading around to the back and the porch. Across from it was an old beaten down shed with a tall oak tree with sprawling branches high up and a tire swing. The garden had been turned over some weeks earlier, and new plants had been put into the soil. The back porch ran the width of the house, with several steps climbing up to it. There was a squeaky sound to the door as it opened and a patio table with chairs sitting atop a green grass carpet. The back door was white, with chipped paint, an old weathered sign over it read *George and Ruby Peirce*. Her grandmother was opening the door as they came up.

"Gram, this is Jeremy, Calvin's friend," Carley said. Jeremy smiled at her and offered his hand which the old woman shook.

"Nice to meet you," Ruby said. "I understand you're going to help with the refrigerator?"

"Yes," Jeremy said, remembering how Calvin had been corrected on the phone.

"Oh, thank you," she said. "Will you be staying for dinner too? I made enough if that's all right."

"That would be great," Jeremy said.

"Now, I understand you're Jewish, but does that mean you can't eat shellfish?" she asked. "I only ask because I made something that had crab meat in it."

"Oh it's fine, Mrs. Peirce," Jeremy said. "I can eat whatever. We had bacon the other day,"

"Carley's eyes widened and she nudged his foot. Feeling the need to clarify, Jeremy added, "At my parent's."

Calvin arrived a few moments later, just as Carley had predicted. There was a half case of Narragansett in one hand and a set of ratchet ties in the other as he stepped into the kitchen.

He went to Ruby, kissing her on the cheek, before brushing up against Carley, knocking her into the wall before he addressed Jeremy.

"You're prompt," Calvin said to him as he set the ratchets on the table. He opened the fridge and set the beer inside, tearing into the box and pulling a pair of cans out, setting one in front of Jeremy. Gram was already on her way to the basement, the light switching on by a pulley string overhead as she began working her way down the steps of the old house.

"Well, let's get this over with," Calvin muttered, following Ruby into the basement. Carley followed from behind grabbing Jeremy's rear as he stepped into the doorway.

The basement was dark and musty, with furniture placed haphazardly around the floor. The furniture looked old, but not terribly out of date. Calvin looked around the place, an old crib leaning against the stone and concrete wall. There was a sadness to the place, and despite the sunlight breaking through the small windows at intervals in the foundation, it seemed dark, yet not uncomfortable.

"It's this one," Ruby explained, putting her hand on the tall refrigerator. It had been in there for years and still worked, apparently only until recently. Calvin had plugged it in from time to time when he's snuck beer into the house. "I guess you'll just take it out the bulkhead. The man said to put it out by the end of the driveway."

"Got it, Gram," Calvin said as he unwound the set of ratchet straps.

"I'll be upstairs finishing dinner," she said as she started making her way back to the stairs. Calvin waited till she was at the top of the stairs before he turned to Jeremy and spoke.

"This was all the stuff from our house in Attleboro," Calvin explained. "All our furniture and things got placed down here when my mom moved out of the house we were renting."

Carley plopped down in an old armchair, pulling her feet up and under her.

"I used to come down here after we visited Mom," Carley said. "This place made her more real somehow. It was like touching the stuff that belonged to her."

"Us," Calvin reminded her. "Anyway, there's a hand truck out in the shed. Can you go get it, Carley?"

"Yup," Carley answered as she got up.

"Bring it around to the bulkhead," Calvin said. "I'll have the doors opened."

Carley climbed the stairs to the kitchen and stepped out onto the linoleum floor. Ruby looked at her from the sink with an expression that said there was something on her mind. She was about to speak when she paused, pointing the short knife in her hand at the cellar door saying,

"Shut the door."

Carley closed it with the palm of her hand, feeling a tingling sensation at the back of her neck and the pit of her stomach suddenly going topsy-turvy. Ruby looked back into the sick and continued working on their dinner.

"I don't know who you think you're fooling," she whispered. "But that's your brother's friend down there."

"We're just friends," Carley whispered back. "It's not like that."

"It's not? Then explain to me what I saw in my front yard five minutes before your brother got here," Ruby said.

"It just happened," Carley said. "But I like him, all right? I shouldn't need Calvin's permission to go out with somebody."

"That doesn't just happen," Ruby corrected her. "I may be old, but I'm not stupid, Carley Louise Peirce." Ruby turned back to her granddaughter, sighed and continued. "But I do approve. He seems like a nice young man."

"He is," Carley agreed.

"Just be respectful of your brother, that's all I have to say about it," Ruby said.

"We haven't said anything to Calvin yet. We wanted him to see how things are with the two of us as friends before we told him. It's important, so please don't say anything."

"Are you spending time with him?" Ruby asked crookedly. She let her stoic Peirce gaze linger on Carley for a moment before she answered.

"Yes," Carley said shortly as she went to the door.

"Well, just be careful," Ruby reminded her.

SECTION VIII

She wasn't sure that it was the best life choice to make, staring at the silver stud that poked out of her upper lip, just below and to the let of her nose. It sparkled and was slightly red around the edges, but she had been cleaning it with a bottle of peroxide that Jeremy had smuggled home from the truck. Using a q-tip, she dabbed the end into the solution and wiped the area around it clean. The sound of the front door opening caught her attention.

Jeremy came in, a heavy cloud hanging over him. Carley picked up on it immediately as he put his hand on the back of her couch. He hadn't told her that he was coming over, and she wasn't expecting him.

"Baby, what is it?" she asked. He had a serious look on his face and for a moment she thought he was about to break off their relationship with her.

"Is anyone else here?" he asked. Carley shook her head, and he broke down. She hurried to him, grabbing his shirt and holding onto him, trying to do anything to stop the flood of emotion, not entirely sure that this wasn't about them. She tried to remember if there was anything she'd done recently that had made him upset, but the way he reached out for her there was no way that he wanted to break anything off with her. He was there because he needed her.

"What's wrong?" she asked.

"I'm off the next three days," he said. "There was a woman. She was pregnant," he tried to continue, but the story was too much for him. He broke down again, and she brought him to the couch, sitting him down.

"She died," Jeremy managed to finish. "Her baby too."

"What the fuck?" was all Carley could manage. She opened her arms and held him.

"Don't tell Calvin about this," Jeremy said. "Please. I don't want him to think I can't handle it."

"Baby, he isn't going to know anything about any of this," Carley hushed. "He already doesn't know about us, so why would I tell him?"

He didn't say much the rest of the night. There was a movie playing, but he wasn't paying much attention. He was processing the emotions in his mind, replaying the moments over and over again on a wicked carousel in his brain. It was all on a loop for him, the sounds, sights, even the smells were there, and he judged himself on all of it, right from start to finish.

"So you care if I stay here tonight?" he asked. "My place is too lonely."

"Of course," Carley said. "I want you here."

He was asleep on the couch before the movie was over. It was a dark kind of sleep as if he hadn't rested in days. There was no dreaming, only the blackness of his mind as his body continued to block out the visions from his experience.

He rolled over, feeling her move as he did. She put her arm around his shoulder.

"Where are you going?" she asked.

"Bathroom?" he asked. He didn't need to go, though. It was a sense of need to move that he couldn't shake. She sat up in bed, pulled her hair behind her ear and let him go if he needed to. Putting his feet on the floor, he stopped and sighed, running his palms over his face.

He was gone in the morning, only a note left on the table written on an unopened bill. He'd gone home to shower and change his clothes. It left her unsettled, because he had left clothes at her place before, and while they were dirty, she could have washed them for him. If there was something she wanted now it was to take care of him. Picking up her cell phone she dialed his number, but it went to voicemail after the fifth ring. An uneasy pit developing in her stomach, she paced around the apartment. She tried to play music to put her mind at ease, but the idea that Jeremy was off somewhere trying to wrestle with something so immense as what he'd described to her left her wondering, admittedly selfishly, if he didn't find comfort in her presence anymore. Would this be the end of them somehow?

Pacing past the front window, she saw Calvin pull up along the sidewalk. Hurriedly she rushed around the apartment, looking for anything that might have told him that Jeremy had been there. Hearing him clomp up the steps she checked herself in the mirror before answering, trying to look as typical of herself as she could. She switched on the stereo in her room to complete the Carley effect and got herself into character.

It was eleven o'clock in the morning and she answered eating her breakfast bowl of macaroni and cheese. Chewing with her mouth open, she waved him in. He looked tired; drained of his normal self. Whatever they'd experienced together, Calvin was no better off than Jeremy was. It was really too late to do anything about it, but she glanced around the apartment a second time, wondering if Jeremy had left anything. She turned to Calvin, swallowed a mouthful of Mac and Cheese and asked,

"I was going to call you. Does this look infected?" she asked pointing to the Munroe piercing. The site was a little pink around the area of the stud, but it wasn't inflamed or draining any kind of fluid or puss.

"Nah it looks okay, how long has it been in there?"

"Just a couple days, but it hurts like hell."

"Of course it does dumb ass, you have a piece of metal stuck in your face. It's going to hurt."

"Don't be an asshole," she said falling into her typical character. It was remarkably hard for her to act naturally with him, and she wondered if Calvin was picking up on her nervousness.

The worst part was that she already knew what was bothering him, but couldn't say so.

"Has Gram seen that yet?"

"No."

"You know she's gonna be pissed."

She didn't care, she was the baby and she knew that Gram would probably give some speech about her beauty and then sigh about how much of a shame it was. Carley walked back into her room plopping down in her desk chair. As soon as she did, she spied the Bristol County EMS shirt that she'd pilfered from Jeremy's bedroom. She stuffed it down between her desk and the wall, hopeful that her brother hadn't seen it. It was time for deflection.

"So what do you want?" she asked putting her feet up onto her unmade bed in the most relaxed way possible. He was welcome in the room, but she was barring his entrance beyond where she sat. Her room was the usual mess with her clothes strewn about the place. Her stereo was in the corner and had two large floor speakers pumping out music. They were stained with ash marks and melted candle wax. A Snow Patrol poster hung over the stereo and the walls were brittle behind a thin layer of faded wallpaper desperately holding back the ancient horsehair plaster. Calvin looked at the floor and studied the stained carpet, and then looked back up to Carley.

"What's your inventory like?"

"What do you want?"

"A dime bag would do it."

She leaned forward and grabbed her glasses off her bedside table. They had thick black frames that she has glued plastic rhinestones to. They looked ridiculous on her, but she liked them so who was he to argue? She knelt down and reached under her bed and pulled out a cigar box and tossed it up on the messy tangle of bedsheets and blankets. Calvin sat down next to it on the bed.

"What gives?" she asked. She looked up at him, wanting Calvin to tell her what she already knew.

"About...?"

"Is there some party you haven't told me about?" she asked him forcing an accusing smile.

"No. Just had a really bad day and I couldn't sleep last night."

She fished out a sandwich bag filled about halfway with bud and tossed it onto his lap. There was also one or two others in the box that looked like they were probably mushrooms. He pulled out his wallet. Calvin was withholding information from her, and it was infuriating. Their grandmother had always said that she wouldn't have said shit if he'd had a mouth full of it, and that was certainly the case now. "What's wrong?" she asked.

"I pretty much had the worst day ever yesterday, and I was up all night because of it."

"What happened?"

He relayed the story of the woman and her unborn child. He tried to start it off vaguely but as it went along he became more and more precise about details and events, feelings and other things. With each sentence it became more and more real to him. She felt terrible, for both her brother and her lover. She swallowed hard, a sense of anxiety over everything that was this awful Jeremy secret starting to boil up. She couldn't tell him she already knew, but worst of all she didn't know what she could say to him about what he'd experienced. She loved her brother and she loved Jeremy. It was then, in the midst of all that pain and anguish, that she realized that she really did. It wasn't just some silly infatuation. She was capable of such feelings and Carley knew that now. She was in love with Jeremy.

Carley looked at him. His face was vacant, like his mind was a thousand miles away. What he needed was a connection to something other than the thoughts and images in his mind. He needed to be brought back to a place where he was loved and protected. A place where he was important and needed. If there was anyone who knew the value of Calvin Peirce, it was his sister Carley.

"Do you remember my doll? Her name was Samantha," Carley asked. Calvin snapped out of his daze and looked at her curiously.

"I think so."

"She had this arm that never stayed on right and would always pop out of the socket."

"Oh yeah. Well, that's because you always carried her around by the arm."

"Yeah well, what about my old bike and how the chain always fell off, and Gram's kitchen cabinets?"

"What about them?"

"You always knew how to fix Samantha's arm so that it wouldn't 'hurt'. You could get the chain to re-loop itself just by turning the pedals, and you could always find the best way to fix the hinges on the doors of the cabinets." She was on a roll now, but she needed to bring it around to the greater point.

"Well, what was I supposed to do? It wasn't like Grampa could do anything about it in Mount Hope Cemetery."

"You did exactly what you were supposed to do," she said. "I grew up believing that if my brother couldn't fix something, it just couldn't be fixed. You knew that there wasn't anything you were going to do for that lady and her baby, but you tried, I know you did. Because that's who you are."

Calvin shrugged. She was right and he knew it. He looked dejected still, but she was glad to have said all those things. Carley knew that she could be as subtle as a hand grenade, but what there was something on her mind she could channel her grandmother Ruby Peirce and push her way through to being heard. In reality there had never been a time when she felt the ability to tell her brother how much he meant to her, and even if she was betraying him with Jeremy somehow, she wanted him to know that he was one of the most important people in her life and that she loved him. Calvin seemed to teeter between what she'd said and wondering about his own part in the matter the day before. He thumbed his nose, looking eagerly at the bag of weed in front of him.

"How's Jeremy holding up?" she asked. He looked at her

crookedly for a moment, and she wondered if she saw suspicion in his eyes. Carley was still worried about him, and the fact that he hadn't picked up when she'd called worried her. "Let me know if you hear from him," she said. Calvin pulled out a few bills and tossed them into the cigar box next to Carley. She tried to give it back to him, but he insisted, pocketing the bag of weed and dragging his feet out the door.

She spent the rest of the morning and early afternoon fussing around the apartment. She tried calling Jeremy again, but he didn't answer.

"Babe," she said leaving a message. "I'm worried about you, and I don't want to sound gay or anything, but I want to hear your voice. Call me please?"

She spent the night waiting for his call, but it never came. He was either avoiding her, or wasn't in a place where he could talk, but her mind went to the idea that he wanted space. Why would he want space from her though? If he'd been so traumatized by something she wanted to console him. She wanted to hold him and tell him that he'd done everything he could and that he was an amazing medic. She wanted him to know that he meant everything to her.

There wasn't much to do, and the night turned into early morning. She drove out to the house in Ocean Grove the next morning. She put on the shirt that had belonged to Jeremy which she'd claimed as her own. It was a little stale smelling, but that didn't mean it wasn't clean. It smelled like him anyway and she wanted that to carry with her.

The tire swing listed gently in the breeze, and like calling her back to her childhood, Carley put her feet through it, testing the rope, and wondering where Jeremy and Calvin were and what they were doing. Her grandmother wasn't home, but she let herself in anyway, heading down into the basement where the couch that had sat in her mother's living room was residing. She dropped down onto it, looking up at the boards above her head and the nails that fastened them to the beams. It was dark and quiet in the basement, a good place to think.

Carley was startled awake by the sound of her phone chiming. She looked around for a moment, before remembering that she was in her grandmother's basement and that she'd gone down there to escape something. She remembered Jeremy and the strange feeling she'd had about the patient he'd lost. Looking at her phone, she had a message from him.

Hey, the text message said.

'Where are you, I'm worried sick about you.'

Sorry, I didn't want to worry you. I'm outside your place, but you're not here.

'I'm at Gram's house,' she replied. 'I'm coming home, don't go anywhere.' She was up immediately and heading for the steps when he answered her.

I'm on my way to Union Hospital for a critical indecent stress debriefing, he explained. *I'll come by later, I promise.*

Carley grit her teeth and climbed the stairs to the kitchen. Ruby was there, sitting at the table with a cup of tea in her hand and she seemed puzzled to see her granddaughter emerging from the basement.

"Hi, Gram," Carley sighed.

"You scared me half to death," Ruby replied. "How long have you been down there?"

Carley shrugged. "I got here this morning and I must have fallen asleep on the couch."

"I wish you wouldn't spend so much time down there," Ruby said. She got up from the table and opened the cabinet taking down a package of cookies. "Would you like some tea?"

Tea was her grandmother's staple, and normally she would have refused, eager to get away from the house and off to something more exciting. The idea of driving away to nothing seemed to bother her more than the notion of a cup of tea with Ruby Peirce though, and she nodded, opening the cabinet beside the stove and pulling down her old mug; the one with a mother duck followed by several ducklings.

"What's wrong?" Gram asked as Carley poured the hot water into her mug from the kettle.

"Something with Jeremy," Carley replied. "Calvin too. They had a bad call the other day and now Jeremy is distant. I've been trying to call him, but he only just now got back to me. He's going to some sort of debriefing at the hospital now."

Ruby nodded, pushing the package of cookies to Carley. She thought for a moment before speaking, dipping her cookie in her tea before chewing it. She brushed the crumbs off her fingers, dabbing then on the napkin beside her.

"When you grandfather was in the war he wrote to me almost every day. I'd get telegrams or letters from him, but he never talked about what he was doing or what he saw. I suppose that he was under orders not to do so, but when he came home it remained the same. He was a different man when he came back. Nervous all the time, and loud noises made him jump. He never talked about the war, except around people who'd been there too. When he got involved with the fire department and the emergency squad I was worried that he would totally close off to me."

Ruby looked out the window, seeing the orange and yellow leaves still attached to the tire swing tree. Her grandfather had hung that tire swing for their mother when she was a little girl, and she and Calvin had used it when they were kids as well. It was one of the things about the house that let them know that George Peirce was still around in his own way.

"It seemed to do him good though. It was a way for him to put his skills to use. He was a lot like your brother, and I know I'm not the first person to say that Calvin took after him. Neither of them would say a damn word about what was on their minds. They're stubborn like that."

Ruby sipped her tea and looked sternly at the new facial jewelry that was on Carley's face. She shook her head, not wanting to address the issue. Carley could have known what she was thinking, that there was no reason to do such a thing when she had such a beautiful face, and even Carley had to admit that it was an impulsive move on her part to get the Munroe. It seemed like such a stupid thing to do now.

"I still think about those letters and telegrams though," Ruby lamented. "For some reason I threw them away. I don't know why I did that. I have things that are his from the war, but those letters would have done more to send me back. I'd be able to hear his voice when I read them. They were his words, and I can't get them back now."

She reached across the table and took Carley's hand, squeezing it, and letting her fingers rest there. The cuff of her sweater pulled back showing the old woman's wrist and the veins that ran along it. Her skin was like paper, but Ruby Peirce was a strong woman.

"Sometimes men need to find ways of dealing with things that they can't explain. Jeremy's a good boy though, I wouldn't worry too much. The strong silent types like your brother, or your grandfather, even Jeremy need to go off and think before they know what to do about bad situations. Give him a little time. He'll come back around."

The sun was going down by the time she got back to her apartment. She pushed the door closed with her sneaker and dropped her keys on the table, heading for the kitchen for a beer. The Peirce House always lacked beer, but if Calvin had been working over there, there might have been some left over. There hadn't been, and now all Carley wanted was to crack one open and wait for another word from Jeremy. As if in answer to her thought, there was a banging on the front door. Looking around the kitchen corner, she could see Jeremy and her brother standing behind the glass, looking disheveled. She ran to the door.

"Oh my God, what happened?!" Carley shrieked opening the door for them. They shuffled their feet in, and Jeremy leaned against the wall while Calvin allowed himself to collapse on her ratty yellow couch. Jeremy's glasses were missing from his face. Calvin's eye was swollen, and his lip was fat. Blood had already dried on his shirt and the skin beneath his lip.

"Little scuffle," Calvin replied.

"Where are your glasses?" Carley asked Jeremy as she looked over his injuries. He winced in pain as she touched his face where Ron had landed his successful blows. "I'll get you some ice," he said. "Sit on the couch," she instructed leading Jeremy there.

She returned a moment later with a pair of ice packs and an old bag of frozen peas. She handed one of the packs to Calvin and all but crawled onto Jeremy's lap to tend to his wounds.

"Oh I'm fine, really," Calvin insisted as Carley ignored him.

"What happened?" Carley demanded. "Are you in trouble?"

"Maybe, I dunno," Jeremy said. Carley groaned sympathetically and removed the ice pack she'd been holding against his face and kissed his swollen eye.

"Poor thing," she said.

"Again, I'm fine," Calvin said. "Please don't make a fuss…"

As if realizing that she'd blown her cover Carley jumped off

Jeremy and corrected her face to one of indifference to him. She was still wearing the shirt that she had stuffed between her desk and the wall, and Calvin could see that it was Jeremy's blue Bristol County shirt. She looked at Jeremy and then back at Calvin in defiance and said

"Well I don't care if you know," she said, feeling a burning rage build up inside her. He had some damn nerve calling her on her sneaking around with his friend. "I'm sick of hiding it, and you're not going to come in here all beaten up and expect me to feel guilty about..."

"I don't care, Carley," Calvin said. "He never said anything, I figured it out for myself. Honestly, I'm happy for you both so... carry on."

Carley sighed and asked Calvin "You need something?"

"A beer would be nice," he said. "I didn't get to finish mine."

Carley returned with three cans of Narragansett, handed one to Calvin and opened the one for Jeremy, leaving her own on the sofa table until she was confident Jeremy was comfortable enough. Calvin was glad to see this, as Carley had never shown this much attention to any guy he'd remembered her going with. She seemed different with him, more adult. She kissed Jeremy again, taking care not to hurt him. "Love you," she whispered to him.

Carley was leaning against Jeremy, her arm wrapped around his. Their hands clasped together in full view of the person they had been so afraid of betraying with their relationship. Calvin cracked the top of his beer and a foamy head billowed onto the top of the can. There hadn't been much said about the issue, and Jeremy supposed that there wasn't a need for it. Calvin wasn't about to lose his cool over his best friend dating his little sister. The revelation of the plot against him from John Prince and Bobby Carreiro had failed, and Calvin wasn't about to sell him, or anyone out, to make his own way easier.

"We'll be sore tomorrow," Calvin remarked as he got up to leave. It was late, and they had one more day off until they were expected back at work. "Tylenol, ice, and ibuprofen," Calvin said. "And beer. Beer fixes everything," he surmised. "Later," he said as he was pushing open Carley's front door.

"You're sure you're all right?" Carley asked Calvin as he made his way through the door. He nodded noncommittally, but Carley was climbing over the top of the couch and into the hall as he let the screen door close behind him. She pushed it open again and rushed out onto the porch. "Hey!" she called after him.

"What?" he asked at the bottom of the steps. He turned around, just a tinge of irritation on his expression.

"You sure you're okay?" she asked. She wasn't asking about his wounds, or even the horrible call they'd run. She was asking about something so personal and important to her. This wasn't some small thing and Calvin knew it. She was serious about this, because there was a look on her face that went well beyond simple infatuation or a passing interest. This was the real thing, and he'd heard her tell Jeremy she loved him.

"I'm okay," he said. "I wish it hadn't been kept a secret for so long, but I'm happy for you."

"You're not mad at him?" she asked. "Or me?"

Calvin shook his head. "Why would I be? Honestly, I think you're good for each other. I think you've probably helped him out of his shell in a way I couldn't. And I think that you might learn a few things from him too."

Carley leaned against the post on the porch, her hands behind her back as she knocked her toe against the aged wood. There was a peculiar feeling she'd had since she'd started dating Jeremy, and even she had to admit that she felt different about herself. What had started out as a curious sort of infatuation had turned into something that she'd never expected from herself.

"Gram seems to like him," Calvin said. "You know Ruby gave him a thorough once over. He seemed to have met her standard." Carley nodded.

"She gave me a ration of shit over it too," Carley said smirking. "I wonder if she thought I wasn't good enough for him."

Calvin shook his head. "You're the baby. Nothing is good enough for *you*."

"But you'll still be cool to him, right?" she asked. "I don't want this to make things weird because of some stupid Bro-Code or something."

Calvin sighed, made the sign of the cross, and reiterated, "You have my blessing."

Carley smirked, the typical curled lip Peirce expression and promptly flipped her brother off. He turned and walked out to the sidewalk, his car waiting for him in the spot where its tires had come to a screeching halt.

Carley ran back into the house. She was about to pounce on Jeremy, but slowed down, crawling up beside him where he sat, laying her head on his lap. His face was still red, and his beer was half gone.

"You want another?" she asked. Jeremy nodded, shaking the can checking to see how much was left. He downed the rest of it in a gulp as Carley got up and went to the kitchen. Watching her go, Jeremy picked up his glasses, holding them together and looking at her through the broken frames. She looked back at him as he was smiling at her, despite his situation.

"I meant it, you know," she said, leaning on the open refrigerator door. He propped the broken glasses on his nose, trying to balance them so he could see. It made her smile, and her point all the more appropriate.

"Meant what?" he asked.

"When I told you I loved you," she said almost immediately ducking into the fridge in case he didn't feel the same way. There was no hesitation, though, and as she came back up with a fresh pair of beers he said,

"I love you too."

Carley bit her lip, the metal of her snake bite rubbing against the enamel of her teeth. Popping the top of the two beers, she tossed the tabs onto the counter top where they rattled against the backsplash before coming to a rest. They were exposed now, what they were was no longer a secret. Her feet caught the rug beneath her and Jeremy grinned, smiling through a swollen lip. Sitting on the couch beside him, she leaned against the arm and passed him his beer. She took a swallow, feeling him lean over her, curling up against her, his head in her lap. It was a quiet moment, without the noise and busyness of her tumultuous life. There was peace here, and happiness. It was like nothing she'd ever experienced before. She stroked his hair with her fingers, feeling the curvature of his ear as they relaxed. Here, in the midst of all the anxiety and chaos of the world, there was peace.

James Windale

ABOUT THE AUTHOR

James Windale is the author of *Twenty-Five at the Lip*, *Bright Lights and Cold Steel*, *Tuesday's Gone*, and *Just Say Maybe*. He also helped co-author *The Delirium: A Zombie Opera of the Great War*, with sci-fi author Jeremy Brinkett. When not writing he works as a paramedic in Florida.

James Windale

www.ingramcontent.com/pod-product-compliance
Lightning Source LLC
Chambersburg PA
CBHW071447180526
45170CB00001B/496